Guide to Federal Pharmacy Law

4th Edition

Barry S. Reiss, Ph.D.
Professor Emeritus
Albany College of Pharmacy
Albany, New York

Gary D. Hall, M.S.
Professor of Pharmaceutics
Albany College of Pharmacy
Albany, New York

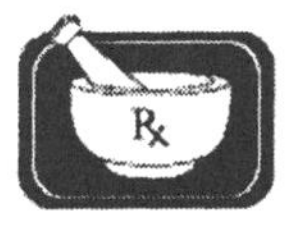

Apothecary Press
Delmar, New York
2005

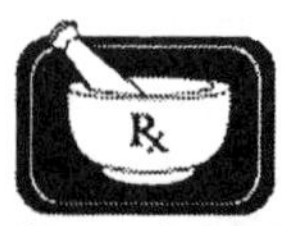

Table of Contents

Preface

On behalf of Apothecary Press and the authors, we welcome you to our Guide to Federal Pharmacy Law, 4th Edition. This Guide has been prepared to assist you in making the review of federal pharmacy law as simple and painless as possible.

The Guide is divided into fourteen sections, each of which is designated with a letter. Within some sections there are sample questions similar to the type that may be seen on the MPJE®. Answers to these questions are provided immediately below the questions. By popular demand, we have added an Index to this edition. This should be a useful tool in helping the reader to easily find specific areas of interest.

At the end of this Guide are close to 300 multiple-choice questions that cover the federal statutes addressed by this book. Candidates are encouraged to attempt to answer these questions only after they have completed studying the contents of this Guide. This will serve as a practice examination that will help to identify areas of weakness that require further study. Answers to these questions may be found at the very end of the question section.

This edition also includes a comprehensive list of names, addresses, phone numbers, and e-mail contacts for each of the state boards of pharmacy in the United States. Candidates are advised to first contact the board of pharmacy in the state(s) in which they plan to seek licensure in order to obtain the latest information about specific state requirements.

Barry S. Reiss
Gary D. Hall

Section A

Guide to the MPJE®

Applying for and Taking the MPJE®

The MPJE® is a computerized law examination, which is required in most states for individuals to obtain a pharmacist license. Pharmacists attempting to reciprocate their licenses to another state are also often required to pass the MPJE®. The examination consists of questions based upon both federal drug laws and regulations and upon the laws and regulations of the specific state.

All candidates are advised to obtain the latest copy of the NAPLEX®/MPJE® Registration Bulletin, which may be downloaded from NABP's website at

www.nabp.net

This bulletin is updated on a regular basis and describes the procedures for applying for and taking the computerized examination.

Remember that each state has established its own criteria for determining a candidate's eligibility to take the MPJE® examination. However, the following guidelines may be useful to simplify the application process:

- Carefully review the NABP®'s Registration Bulletin because changes may be made to the guidelines at any time.

- Complete the registration form and mail it to your STATE BOARD OF PHARMACY with the required fees. Be sure to apply for the appropriate examination (i.e. either the NAPLEX® or the MPJE®).

- Your state's board of pharmacy will notify NABP® of your eligibility to take the examination.

- If you are qualified to take an examination, an Authorization to Test (ATT) will be sent to you. It will indicate the dates of your eligibility, an ATT number, a candidate identification number, and an expiration date (usually about 1 year).

- You may contact any testing center location to schedule your individual testing time. Presently Prometric testing centers are being used. When contacting the testing site, have the following available:

    - authorization number
    - candidate ID number
    - expiration date from your ATT card

- Arrive at the testing center at least 15 minutes early. Have available:
  - your ATT
  - two forms of identification, at least one of which must have a picture ID with signature. (Driver's license or passport is acceptable)
- The computerized examination must be completed in two hours. Extra time will be provided to complete a questionnaire and a short tutorial.

- No food, drink, reference books, or notes are allowed.

- You are not permitted to open personal belongings such as bags or wallets during the exam.

- Your examination score will be reported only to the board of pharmacy of the state you have designated.

Content of the MPJE®

The MPJE® examination will most likely consist of 90 multiple-choice questions of which 60 will contribute to your score. The remaining 30 are intermingled throughout the exam and are "pretest questions". That is, they are new questions, which the NABP® is evaluating for level of difficulty and appropriateness. Some of these may show up in later examinations as questions that will count!

The level of difficulty for MPJE® questions will vary. While the passing score for the exam is set at 75, it does NOT mean that you have to correctly answer at least 75% of the questions in order to pass. The actual number of correct answers needed to pass a specific examination will vary from one exam to another.

The person next to you may have some test questions that are different from yours in wording, topics covered, and degree of difficulty. The cardinal rule to remember is simply to answer ALL questions to the best of your ability. Do not become discouraged if you have several very difficult questions.

The examination will have questions involving federal laws and regulations as well as specific state laws and regulations. The questions will be intermingled. Clearly, you should be familiar with not only the federal laws and regulations, but also those of the state to which you are applying. Because each state has its own unique laws, this Guide is focused only on federal laws and regulations.

MPJE® Competency Statements

The NABP® has established a set of competency statements designed to acquaint the candidate with the topics that may be included on the examination. The MPJE® Bulletin describes the three major areas included in the examination. These consist of:

Area 1   **Pharmacy Practice** (approximately 78 % of the exam)

Area 2   **Licensure, Registration, Certification, and Operational Requirements** (approximately 17 % of the exam)

Area 3   **Regulatory Structure and Terms** (approximately 5% of exam)

The candidate may wish to review the competencies listed under each of the above areas. However, the statements are not very descriptive. Obviously the examination will stress those laws and regulations with which any individual entering the profession should be familiar. These will include:

- Requirements for obtaining and maintaining a pharmacist license including continuing education (CE) requirements.

- The structure and duties of a board of pharmacy and authorized inspection bodies.

- The standards of practice for both the filling and refilling of prescriptions.

- Individual state requirements for drug substitution.

- Procedures for the purchase, storage, and record keeping of drugs.

- Regulations for counseling of patients and guaranteeing the confidentiality of their prescriptions and medical records.

- Requirements for the registration and maintenance of a pharmacy whether in a community or institutional setting.

- Additional requirements for the purchase, storage, record keeping, and dispensing of controlled substances.

- The pathways and requirements for bringing new drugs to the market.

- Individual laws and regulations, of either state or federal origin, which impact upon the practice of pharmacy (e.g. Orphan Drug Act).

While some of the above concepts are described in individual state law, many are under the jurisdiction of federal agencies; for example, the labeling of OTC's (nonprescription drugs), dietary and nutritional supplements, and cosmetics.

Study Tip

Obviously you must review both the federal and your specific state's pharmacy laws since approximately 50% of your exam will be based upon state law. This review book is intended to concentrate on federal pharmacy law, which is appropriate for all states.

It is the objective of this book to review material most likely to be on your exam. Naturally there will always be a few questions from "left field" that were neither presented in this Guide or in your pharmacy college's Jurisprudence course. Don't worry about the isolated facts. Instead, concentrate on major topics. You are fortunate if you are taking the exam in a state that closely follows federal law.

Study Tips

In reviewing for the exam, your objective is to learn the law and to recognize what areas of the law are applicable in a particular question. DO NOT attempt to memorize the exact citation for a law such as 503; 21 U.S.C. 353 for the Durham-Humphrey Amendment or a state regulation designation such as "Section 2857" of the Public Health Law. While it may be useful to learn the date of origin for major laws such as the FD&C Act of 1938, it is very unlikely that you will be specifically questioned on the dates of less significant legislation.

Remember also that when legislation is passed, it may not immediately take effect. For example, the Durham-Humphrey Amendment was passed by Congress in 1951 but did not become effective until 1952.

Spend most of your review time on questions related to the federal Controlled Substances Act. Obviously it is also important to concentrate on your individual state's pharmacy laws and regulations.

When reviewing specific laws and regulations, carefully note the difference between the designations of "shall" and "may". The term "shall" like the term "must" is an absolute requirement. The term "may" is looser, indicating the permission to do something. For example, the pharmacist shall place poison prevention closures on prescription containers versus the pharmacist may supply prescription package inserts to a patient when dispensing a drug.

Tips for Answering MPJE® Questions

Questions on the MPJE® are likely to be in one of two formats. Many questions will have a simple stem followed by five choices lettered A through E. The candidate must select the BEST answer and key that answer into the computer. Other questions will be in the format known as multi-response questions, combined response, or "K" questions. These simply refer to questions with a simple stem followed by three choices numbered I, II, and III. The answer choices will consist of several single and combinations of these three choices. The format always used for answer choices in "K" questions is:

(A)   I only
(B)   III only
(C)   I and II only
(D)   II and III only
(E)   I, II, and III

"K" questions are frequently found on the NAPLEX® and, to a lesser extent, on the MPJE®. These questions are usually considered to be more difficult than standard multiple-choice questions since the candidate is not just seeking a single correct answer but possible combinations of correct answers. While many federal laws and regulations are complex, MPJE® examiners are generally realistic and are unlikely to ask the candidate to identify obscure facts about federal laws.

> ## Study Tip
>
> When answering a "K" question, ignore the combinations of answers until you have closely evaluated each choice. For each, decide if it is true or correct, and then hope that your answer among the choices offered. For example, if you decide that I and II are correct answers and III is not, obviously you would key in (C) as the answer. However if you have selected the combination of I and III, you will quickly notice that this combination is not in the answer key. Obviously you should reconsider as to whether just I or III are correct or if it is possible that II is also correct? A second situation occurs when you have decided that III is correct, I is not correct, but you are uncertain about choice II. It is probably better to go with what you know to be correct, i.e., the choice of III only.

Other things to remember while you are taking the MPJE® include:

- Read each question carefully and try to determine what concept, general principle or specific law is being tested. Remember that when there is a conflict between federal and an individual state's law, the stricter usually applies (e.g. if a controlled drug is federally classified in Schedule III and is classified by the state as a Schedule II drug, the more stringent state law applies)

- When a question mentions a specific drug, try to classify it in your mind as a controlled substance, non-controlled prescription-only drug or OTC.

- Assume that each question is written in a straight-forward manner. The examiners are not out to trick you.

- After deciding upon the correct response, complete the answering process using three steps.

  1. Highlight the answer on the computer screen.
  2. Request the next question by keying the icon on the lower right portion of the screen.
  3. Confirm that you want the next question by keying the icon next to the above icon.

Note

Remember that once you have completed steps 2 and 3, you are not permitted to return to the previous question and change your answer. Don't hurry through questions and risk a quick decision. You have plenty of time to complete the examination. On the other hand, don't overanalyze the questions. Your first choice is probably the best choice.

Scoring of your MPJE® is done very quickly and the results are sent to the board(s) of pharmacy you have designated. Remember that you have no way of knowing how well you are doing during the exam. Do not become discouraged if you run into several difficult questions. Simply answer ALL questions to the best of your ability and knowledge. While the passing grade is set at 75%, this does not mean that you have to correctly answer a minimum of 75% of the questions. It is possible that a raw score of below 75% will convert into a passing grade.

Common Errors Made By Candidates

- *Not reading the question carefully*

  Example: Which one of the following is NOT required to be placed by the pharmacist onto a prescription?

  vs.

  Which one of the following is NOT required to be placed by the pharmacist onto a prescription label?

- *Basing your answers on your knowledge of local laws or regulations.*

  Example: Expiration dating on prescription labels is NOT required by either federal or most state laws but may be a local requirement.

- *Basing your answers on what you do in the pharmacy you are employed in.*

  Unfortunately, some pharmacies do not follow the letter of the law. Using your pharmacy's current practice as a guideline for choosing your answer may result in incorrect answers on this examination.

- *Attempting to base an answer on recent changes in the law.*

  New laws or regulations may be ambiguous or poorly understood by practitioners. For this reason, questions on the MPJE® exam are usually based on well established laws and regulations. If a question is based on a fairly recent law it is likely to be a question that is being tested by NABP® and will likely not count toward your score.

Section B

Sources of Laws, Rules and Regulations

Introduction

Many laws and amendments that have shaped the current Food, Drug and Cosmetic Act were enacted over the past 100 years. In most cases they represent attempts on the part of lawmakers to protect the American public.

Pure Food and Drug Act of 1906

Up to 1906 there were relatively few controls on the distribution of foods, drug-containing products, cosmetic products and medical devices. Products were often contaminated, were not consistent in strength and were poorly labeled. In 1906 Congress passed the Pure Food and Drug Act. This law prohibited foods and drugs that were distributed through interstate commerce to be adulterated or misbranded. The law fell short of protecting the public since it did not require manufacturers to list ingredients or directions for use of a product on the label. The law also did not regulate cosmetic products or medical devices.

Food, Drug and Cosmetic Act of 1938

In 1937, 107 deaths caused by the mistaken use of diethylene glycol (automobile anti-freeze), as a vehicle in a sulfanilamide elixir resulted in the passage of a landmark piece of federal regulation, the Food, Drug and Cosmetic Act (FDCA) of 1938. The law required, for the first time in the US, that any new drug could not be marketed unless it had first been proven to be safe when used according to directions on the label. It also required that labels include adequate directions for use and warnings about habit-forming drugs that were contained in the product. It was also the first law that applied to cosmetic products and medical devices as well as to food and drug products.

Drug products marketed prior to 1938 were exempted or "grandfathered" from the law and did not, therefore, have to be labeled or proven safe under this law. The FDCA became the backbone of many subsequent laws and amendments that further strengthened drug control in the US.

Note

Several drug products still sold in pharmacies (e.g. levo-thyroxine, digoxin, nitroglycerin, and phenobarbital) were on the market prior to 1938 and are, therefore, still "grand-fathered" from this law.

Durham-Humphrey Amendment of 1951

Many of the drug products covered by the 1938 FDCA Act were not safe to use without medical supervision. The Durham-Humphrey Amendment of 1951 was enacted to further regulate these products. This was an amendment to the FDCA that established two classes of drugs. Those that required medical supervision to be used safely did not have to list "adequate directions for use" but were required to include the legend "Caution: Federal law prohibits dispensing without a prescription" on the manufacturer's label.

The requirement for "adequate directions for use" was satisfied by the pharmacist placing on the label of the dispensed product, directions provided by the prescriber (e.g. Take one tablet twice daily). Such products became known as prescription or "legend" drugs. Products that did not require medical supervision for their use had to have adequate directions for use on their label and were referred to as "over-the-counter" or nonprescription drug products. In addition to distinguishing between legend and nonprescription drug products, this legislation also provided for oral prescriptions and prescription refills.

Kefauver-Harris Amendment of 1962

The Kefauver-Harris Amendment was adopted as a result of public concern about thalidomide, a tranquilizer drug marketed primarily in Europe. This drug was marketed in Europe but was not approved by the FDA for the US market. In 1961, it was determined that thalidomide had caused serious birth defects in the offspring of many women in Europe who had used the drug.

While there were few birth defects seen in the US, Congress enacted the Kefauver-Harris Amendment to protect the public in the future. This amendment to the FDCA Act (also referred to as the Drug Efficacy Amendment) required that all new drugs marketed in the US had to be shown to be not only safe but also effective. This requirement was also extended to products that had been approved between 1938 and 1962.

In addition to this efficacy requirement, the amendment also included provisions that placed the authority for regulating prescription drug advertising into the hands of the FDA. It also required informed consent for individuals who were research subjects in clinical investigations, reporting of adverse drug reactions, and creation of Good Manufacturing Practice (GMP) requirements that clearly defined the conditions under which drugs could be manufactured in the US.

Medical Device Amendment of 1976

In order to protect the American public against potentially dangerous or useless medical devices, Congress enacted the Medical Device Amendment of 1976. This amendment to the FDCA Act provides for better classification of medical devices according to their specific function, establishment of performance standards for these devices, pre-market approval requirements, conformance with GMP standards, and requirements for adherence to record and reporting requirements.

Orphan Drug Act of 1983

Orphan drugs are those that are used to treat diseases that relatively rare, i.e. they affect relatively few people. Prior to 1983 the cost of developing and marketing such drugs was prohibitive for most drug manufacturers because of their limited potential for profitability. In 1983 Congress enacted the Orphan Drug Act. This provided various tax and licensing incentives to manufacturers that made development of such drugs more appealing. A rare disease is usually considered one that affects less than 200,000 persons in the United States.

Drug Price Competition and Patent-Term Restoration Act

This piece of legislation, sometimes called the Waxman-Hatch Amendment, attempted to resolve a dispute between generic drug and brand name drug manufacturers. Prior to the enactment of this amendment to the FDCA, generic drug manufacturers had to go through most of the lengthy drug approval process that was required of manufacturers of newly developed drugs. New drug manufacturers were concerned about limited periods of exclusive patent rights for their innovative products. In enacting this bill, Congress streamlined the drug approval process for generic products and provided innovative drug manufacturers with incentives to develop new drug products. For example, the "pioneer" drug firm has five years of patent restoration or at least five years of exclusive marketing once a drug has been approved by the FDA.

Prescription Drug Marketing Act of 1987

This bill was enacted in order to place more stringent controls on the distribution of prescription drug samples and to prevent hospitals and other health care entities from reselling pharmaceuticals to other businesses. It was an attempt to more precisely manage the drug distribution system in the US.

FDA Modernization Act of 1997

This Act is a far-reaching piece of legislation that touches virtually every aspect of FDA's activities. Included in this legislation are:

- Provisions for the fast-track review of some New Drug Application submissions. The intent is to expedite the approval of new drugs used to treat serious or life-threatening conditions.

- Clarification of the conditions under which pharmacies may perform extemporaneous compounding of prescriptions. One premise is that individual states should regulate compounding. Also, pharmacies are exempt from the strict regulatory federal GMP standards and the requirements for submission of new drug applications.

- The prescription drug legend "Caution: Federal law prohibits dispensing without a prescription" is replaced by "Rx only".

- The provision that required certain substances to be labeled "Warning – May be habit forming." has been eliminated.

- Encouragement for manufacturers to conduct research for new uses of drugs and to submit supplemental NDA's for these uses. The manufacturers may publicly disseminate limited information about these unapproved uses provided a statement is included specifying that the use has not been approved or cleared by the FDA.

Medicare Modernization Act of 2003

The Medicare Prescription Drug, Improvement and Modernization Act of 2003, commonly referred to as the Medicare Modernization Act (MMA), is a complicated act that was signed into law in December 2003, with some provisions going into effect immediately while others begin in 2006.

In 2004, Medicare beneficiaries, except those under Medicaid may enroll in a Medicare-endorsed, privately run prescription drug discount card program. With an enrollment charge of $30.00, eligible participants may save 10 to 25% of their total drug costs by using this card.

Pharmacies providing services under this program are known as card sponsors and can limit the drug choices available to patients by establishing formularies which must include at least one drug from each of 209 therapeutic categories commonly needed by Medicare beneficiaries. The patient is required to choose a card sponsor from a list of available pharmacies, presumably based upon the location and prices charged by the pharmacy. Once a patient chooses a Medicare-endorsed discount card pro-

Sponsors will probably be able to reduce their drug costs from manufacturers by obtaining drug volume discounts. While they are not required to pass these lower prices to their clients, it is expected that competitive marketplace dynamics will encourage such action.

Low-income families will also receive a subsidy up to $600 a year credited to their drug card. To qualify for such subsidies, current income ceilings are $12,124 for individuals and $16,363 for married couples.

The second phase of the MMA begins in 2006 with a new "Part D" component of Medicare. This benefit will include the cost of any prescription drug, biological product, or insulin, if presently covered by Medicaid and if it is for a medically accepted indication. The premium for this voluntary Part D will be approximately $420 per year ($35/month) and include a $250 annual deductible. Also, the beneficiary will be required to pay for prescription drugs based upon the following sliding scale:

- 25% of their annual drug cost for total expenditures between $251 to $2,250.
- 100% of their annual drug cost for total expenditures between $2,251 to $5,100.

When the beneficiary reaches a total drug expenditure of over $5,100, MMA will again cover them with a co-payment of only $2 for each generic drug prescription filled and $5 for each brand-name prescription filled, or a minimum charge of 5% of prescription price. This $5,100 per year figure is sometimes referred to as the "catastrophic threshold" while the $2,251 to $5,100 gap, where the threshold" while the $2,251 to $5,100 gap, where the patient pays all costs plus the $420 annual premium, is known as the "donut hole".

The following are other MMA provisions:

1. Drug plan sponsors may not require beneficiaries to obtain their prescriptions through mail-order pharmacies.

2. Larger quantities of medication, including 90-day supplies of long-term use drugs, may be obtained at the participating local pharmacy.

3. If a brand-name product is dispensed, the patient must be informed of the availability of a lower-cost generic product..

4. Pharmacists may be eligible to receive payment from Medicare for providing medication therapy management if the client is enrolled in Medicare Part D.

5. Each drug plan sponsor must establish medication therapy management programs for individuals enrolled in Part D of Medicare, if they have multiple chronic conditions such as asthma, diabetes, hypertension, or hyperlipidemia.

6. MMA permits importation of drug products from Canada and some other countries if the HHS certifies that the importation poses no additional risk to the public health.

7. The Act explicitly blocks the use of Medicare's purchasing power to negotiate prices with pharmaceutical manufacturers to obtain lower-cost drugs for the elderly and disabled.

8. Brings higher reimbursement prices paid by Medicare into a lower range. The manufacturer-reported "AWP" will be phased out in favor of an "ASP" – average sales price. This value will be between the actual acquisition price paid and the present AWP.

9. Prevents pharmaceutical companies from filing multiple 30-month stays to prevent competing companies from marketing a generic version of their drug product.

10. Allows multiple manufacturers of a generic product to obtain a 180 day exclusivity period if they file their applications on the first day of eligibility.

Items 9 and 10 are intended to close loopholes in the Drug Price Competition and Patent-Term Restoration Act of 1984 (Waxman-Hatch Amendment) discussed in Section B.

The future of the MMA will depend on the fiscal experience gained during the first year or two of its implementation and by changes made by Congress and other administrative bodies over the next several years. The student is urged to review current information sources to remain abreast of these changes.

Official Compendia

- **United States Pharmacopoeia/National Formulary (USP/NF)**

The US government does NOT publish this reference. It is published by a private organization known as the US Pharmacopoeia Convention (USPC). The *USP/NF* contains monographs of recognized drugs that include their chemical characteristics and standards of quality. Proposed changes in revisions of the USP/NF are published in The Pharmacopoeia Forum (PF), a bimonthly publiccation. While printed as one bound book, the USP and NF are still considered to be two separate entities.

- ***Homeopathic Pharmacopoeia of the United States (HPUS)***

  This is also published by a private organization or convention that updates information concerning homeopathic products or remedies on a regular basis.

<table>
<tr><td align="center">

Note

If a drug is listed by its official name in the USP/NF or HPUS, it must meet the requirements specified in either book. Otherwise, it must have the designation "not USP/NF". Without this designation the drug is considered to be either misbranded or adulterated. If a drug is official in both the USP and HPUS, it must meet the standards established in the USP monograph unless it is distinctly marketed and labeled as a homeopathic drug.

</td></tr>
</table>

Section C

Acronyms and Definitions

The pharmacist is expected to have a working knowledge of health care terminology. It is, therefore, frustrating when one encounters an unfamiliar abbreviation or acronym. Throughout this Guide, we will use such abbreviations or acronyms. The following table will be a useful guide to those most popularly used:

<table>
<tr><td>

Study Tip

Fortunately, the MPJE® is a multiple-choice exam so that you will not likely be asked to give the name of the organization with the acronym "HCFA". However, a question could be worded: "What federal organization is responsible for administering Medicare?" Another question might be "Which Federal department is responsible for the DEA?" (The Department of Justice). It is probably sufficient if you review the following list and simply be able to recognize the meaning of these common acronyms. It is unlikely that any deliberate "trick" question will be asked, such as "Is HCFA an administration or an agency?"

</td></tr>
</table>

Acronyms

AAC

Actual acquisition cost - the actual price a pharmacist pays when purchasing units of a drug product. This price usually represents a discounted price from the average wholesale price (AWP).

ADE or ADR

Adverse drug experience or adverse drug Reaction.

ATF

Alcohol, Tobacco, and Firearms agency.

AWP

Average wholesale price – a published wholesale price for a drug that can be used as the basis for pricing prescription drugs. Usually pharmacies are able to purchase the drug at lower (discounted) prices from the AWP.

CDC

Centers for Disease Control

CFR

Code of Federal Regulations – a compilation of final regulations and notices promulgated by the federal government; published annually by the US Government Printing Office; the above regulations and notices are first published in the Federal Register, a daily publication.

CPSC

Consumer Product Safety Commission

DEA Drug Enforcement Administration - administration responsible for the Federal Controlled Substances Act; part of the U.S. Department of Justice.

DHHS Department of Health and Human Services - department which includes the Food and Drug Administration (FDA).

DME Durable Medical Equipment – equipment that meets three standards:
1. It can stand repeated use
2. It is primarily for a medical purpose (i.e., it is not useful to a person if they have no illness or injury)
3. It is appropriate for use in the home

Examples of DME's include wheelchairs, oxygen tanks, and walkers.

DRG's Diagnosis-related groups - a classifycation system for hospital inpatients based on the principal diagnosis; reimbursement is usually based on days of stay.

DUR Drug utilization review – a review of prescription drug use, prescribing patterns or drug utilization by patients. Its purpose is to determine if appropriate drugs are being prescribed and if those drugs are being used appropriately.

EAC Estimated acquisition cost – an estimated cost of a drug based upon information collected by the DHHS (Dept. of Health and Human Services). Such costs are often based upon quantity purchased.

FDA   Food and Drug Administration

FDCA   Food, Drug and Cosmetic Act
(FD & C Act or FDCA)

FTC   Federal Trade Commission –
responsible for investigating unfair
business practices including misleading
advertising, etc.

GMP   Good Manufacturing Practice

GRAS   Generally recognized as safe –
refers to a large number of relatively inert
ingredients that are permitted to be used
in pharmaceutical and food products as
excipients or adjuvants because of their
relatively high degree of safety.

GRASE   Generally recognized as safe and
effective - term usually used when
considering nonprescription products.

HCFA   Health Care Financing Administration –
responsible for policies relating to
Medicare (federally managed) and
Medicaid (controlled by individual states
under the supervision of HCFA).

HHA   Home health agency – an organization
licensed or certified by the government to
provide home health care.

HIPAA	Health Insurance Portability and Accountability Act
HMO	Health maintenance organization
HP or HPUS	*Homeopathic Pharmacopoeia of the United States*
HSD	Home-use sterile drug products
JCAHO	Joint Commission on Accreditation Of Health Care Organizations
MAC	Maximum Allowable Cost – the highest price allowed under a specific plan for a specific drug (usually multi-source drugs). If a person wants a more expensive version, he/she must pay the difference.
NABP	National Association of Boards of Pharmacy (create the NAPLEX® and MPJE®).
NDC	National Drug Code – a classification system for identifying a specific drug product; used nationally for reimbursement and for identification of drug products.
NIH	National Institutes of Health
OBRA	Omnibus Budget Reconciliation Act - acts passed each year by Congress for funding many activities; each OBRA known by the year it is enacted.

OSHA   Occupational Safety and Health Administration - monitors work environment to assure worker safety.

OTC   Over-the-Counter - refers to drugs and drug products, which are available without a prescription; also referred to as "nonprescription drug".

PBM   Pharmacy benefits manager

PHS   Public Health Service

PI   Package insert

PPI   Patient package insert

PPO   Preferred Provider Organization – a group of health professionals who are contractually favored to provide health services to individuals under a specific insurance plan.

PPPA   Poison Prevention Packaging Act

SDA   Specially Denatured Alcohol

SNF   Skilled nursing facility - a site that treats patients especially in need of rehabilitation or a lower level of medical care than is needed in a hospital.

TRP   Tamper Resistant Packaging

USAN United States Adopted Names

USP/NF *United States Pharmacopoeia/National Formulary*

USP DI *United States Pharmacopoeia Dispensing Information* - a set of three volumes containing a variety of information. They include

- *Volume I - Drug Information for the Health Care Professional* - contains information about individual drugs. It is written specifically for health professionals.

- *Volume II - Advice for the Patient* – contains drug information in lay language - includes information intended for the general public about the use of drugs, side effects, etc; individual pages may be photocopied and given to patients as part of the counseling process.

- *Volume III - Approved Drug Products With Therapeutic Equivalence Evaluations* – contains information from the Orange Book, USP definitions and regulations, portions of the Federal Controlled Substances Act, plus other information.

Definitions

Cosmetic   Article intended to be rubbed, poured, sprinkled, sprayed on, introduced into or otherwise applied to the human body for the purpose of cleansing, beautifying, promoting attractiveness, or altering the appearance. Also, any component of the above articles is considered to be a cosmetic.

> # Note
> There is one exception to the above –
> Soap is not considered to be a cosmetic.

Device   Any instrument, apparatus, implement, machine, contrivance, implant, *in vitro* reagent or related article which is

- Recognized in the USP/NF or HP or any supplement

- intended for use in the diagnosis, cure, mitigation, treatment, or prevention of disease in man or other animals

- intended to affect the structure or any function of the body of humans or animals but are not foods

> # Note
> Examples of devices would include infusion pumps, cardiac pacemakers and heart monitors.

Drug

1. Article recognized in the official *United States Pharmacopoeia* (USP/NF) official *National Formulary* (NF), or official *Homeopathic Pharmacopoeia of the United States (HPUS),* or any supplements of these references.

2. Article intended for use in the diagnosis, cure, mitigation, treatment, or prevention of disease in man or other animals.

3. Article (other than food) intended to affect the structure or any function of the body of man or other animals

4. Article intended for use as a component of any articles specified in the above but does not include devices or their components, parts, or accessories.

Drug sample

A unit of drug product not intended to be sold. Usually it is intended to acquaint a prescriber with a drug product by providing several doses for short-term or initial therapy.

Food

An article used for food or drink in humans or animals, chewing gum, and substances used as components of food or drink.

> ## Note
> It is unlikely that questions concerning subtle distinctions between foods, drugs, and cosmetics will be asked since there have been too many court decisions and changing opinions that cloud these distinctions. For example, minor claims for "anti-aging" creams have been accepted for cosmetic status while other creams containing hormones are considered to be drug products. Also, some chemicals with therapeutic uses have been classified as dietary supplements.

Generic name — A name that is assigned to a specific drug structure. It is a simplified name as compared to the chemical name. Drug products may be marketed under their "generic name" or a brand name (trade name). The overall implication is that a drug marketed under its generic name only is less expensive than the brand name product.

Hospice — A facility or program that provides palliative and supportive care for terminally ill patients.

Section D

Bringing New Drugs to Market

Investigational New Drug Application (IND)

Before a new drug is marketed, a sponsor (usually a manufacturer) has to complete an extensive testing process to assure that the new drug will be safe and effective for what it is claimed to do. The Investigational New Drug Application (IND) is the first application form that a sponsor must submit to the FDA before a drug may be administered to humans. The requirement for an IND approval is intended to protect both the rights and safety of humans upon whom the drug will be tested.

While most IND sponsors are pharmaceutical companies, it is possible for a medical researcher, academic personnel, or organizations, either public or private, to submit INDs. Once submitted, the FDA has 30 days in which to decide whether the investigational drug is suitable for testing.

Virtually all of the information collected by the sponsor, especially from preclinical (animal) studies, which reflect on both the use and safety of the proposed investigational drug, is submitted to the FDA as part of the IND application. In addition, the sponsor must provide complete descriptions of the methodology (clinical protocols) to be used in testing the drugs in humans.

Clinical Trials

After the FDA approves an IND, the sponsor may initiate clinical (human) trials. There are three phases before the final approval of the drug is provided, and one additional phase after the drug product has been marketed. The drug must satisfactorily complete each phase before it can progress to the next.

- Phase 1   A small group of healthy individuals is given the drug. The primary purpose of this phase is to evaluate the drug's toxicological, pharmacokinetic and pharmacological properties, as well as to assess the safety of the drug in humans.

- Phase 2   A larger group (100 or more) of patients that have the disease or symptoms of the condition to be treated by the drug is given the new drug. The purpose of this phase is to determine the effectiveness of the drug and to obtain information about adequate dosage, relative safety, and adverse effects.

- Phase 3   Large groups of patients (sometimes thousands) in several geographical locations are part of controlled clinical studies. The purpose of this phase is to obtain data concerning the drug's effectiveness as compared to a control group that receives a placebo. Most Phase 3 studies are double-blinded (i.e. neither the patient or investigator knows whether the drug or placebo is being given until after the study is completed)

Phase 1 and 2 studies are usually conducted under the direct supervision of the sponsoring company while Phase 3 studies usually involve testing performed at remote and varied clinical sites by independent investigators. Obviously Phase 3 studies are the most costly and take an extended period of time to complete. In each of these first three phases the patient or their representative must provide informed consent, i.e. they must agree to be subjects in the testing program after having been advised of the potential risks.

Treatment Investigational New Drugs

Treatment INDs allow the administration of an investigational new drug to patients that have not been enrolled in the new drug's clinical trials program. These patients must be in an imminent life-threatening stage of an illness for which there is presently no cure or where the presently used drugs do not appear to be effective. Examples of such diseases might be advanced stages of AIDS, some cancers, Alzheimer's disease, and Parkinson's disease.

The company developing the drug must have presented data outlining the drug's safety and efficacy, and the drug must be in either Phase 2 or 3 of clinical trials. If the drug is being considered as a Treatment IND candidate, a "treatment protocol" must be submitted to the FDA, which describes its proposed use in the designated patients.

The New Drug Application (NDA) Process

Once sufficient data concerning drug efficacy, toxicity, stability, production methods, packaging and the data from numerous clinical trials on patients have been collected, a new drug application may be submitted to the FDA for review. If the FDA reviewers are satisfied with the accuracy and completeness of the data from the clinical trials (Phases 1, 2 and 3), the NDA is approved and the NDA will be "on file" at the FDA. At this point, the manufacturer may market the new drug product.

The NDA often consists of thousands of pages of data and information and is very costly and time-consuming to prepare. Once submitted, the FDA generally reviews the application for at least six months and provides experts and other interested parties the opportunity to comment on the submission.

After the drug product is marketed, Phase 4 studies are conducted. This is the post-marketing surveillance of the drug. During this period, health professionals are encouraged to report any problems with the drug, especially adverse effects experienced when the drug is used. The drug manufacturer must also submit yearly reports concerning new information and field reports concerning the drug product. The FDA utilizes Phase 4 data to determine whether or not a product should remain on the market.

Fast Track Products

A sponsor of a potentially new drug may facilitate its development and review by requesting that the Secretary of the HHS grant it "fast track" status. Generally such status is granted to a product if it is intended for treatment of a serious or life-threatening condition and addresses an unmet medical need. The sponsor must agree to conduct further post-approval studies to validate the product's use.

Abbreviated New Drug Application (ANDA)

Before any new drug may be placed on the market, the innovator company must submit the data described for IND's and NDA's. Usually the innovator pharmaceutical company will have patent protection for their drug entity. However, once the patent expires, other companies may wish to introduce the drug under the drug's generic name only or as a brand name product. Rather than requiring the secondary companies to submit a complete NDA, the FDA will permit an Abbreviated New Drug Application (ANDA) to be submitted. These submissions require less data, but do require proof that the new drug product's pharmacokinetic properties, its bioavailability, and clinical activity is similar to that of the innovator's drug product.

Supplemental New Drug Application (SNDA)

After marketing a drug product, the manufacturer may desire to make some changes in the drug's synthesis, production procedures or manufacturing locations, packaging, labeling, etc. Rather than submit an NDA, the company may submit a Supplemental New Drug Application (SNDA). This abbreviated application permits desired changes to be implemented.

> ## Note
> To distinguish between the necessity for an ANDA versus a SNDA, just picture that any changes or additions made by the company that filed the original NDA will probably require a Supplemental New Drug Application. Examples would include adding a new dosage form, tablet strength, or therapeutic use for the original drug. However if another company is submitting data for a drug product similar to the drug in the original NDA, it will most likely need to file an Abbreviated New Drug Application.

FDA Classification System for New Drugs

During the drug approval process, the FDA classifies new drugs based on their chemical and therapeutic characteristics. Health professionals employ these ratings to assess the potential value of a new drug.

Therapeutic classification

- Type P   Indicates that the drug represents a major therapeutic gain because there are no other effective drugs available for treating a particular illness or because it has significant advantages compared to currently marketed drugs. Drugs classified as Type P are often given a priority review. (Hint: Think "P" = priority)

- Type S   Indicates that the drug is similar to other drugs on the market. Such drugs will generally undergo a standard review. (Hint: Think "S" = standard)

Note

A Type P drug will be reviewed faster than a Type S drug and will, therefore, generally be marketed sooner, if approved by the FDA.

Chemical classification

- Type 1   Indicates a new molecular structure, different from existing drugs, that may be used for the same therapeutic purpose. The drug must not be presently marketed in the United States.

- Type 2   Indicates that the drug is a new derivative of a molecular structure already approved in the United States; for example a new salt or ester of an existing drug.

- Type 3   Indicates that the drug is a new formulation of a drug already marketed in the US.

- Type 4   Indicates that the product is a new combination of two or more drugs.

- Type 5   Indicates that a drug is being manufactured by a new company.

- Type 6   Indicates a new therapeutic indication for a drug already approved.

Note

It is probably NOT necessary to memorize the six chemical classification types. Instead, just remember that Type 1 is the best type since you are placing a new, unique drug on the market. Also remember that Type 6 is important since it will increase the sales and use of a drug product already on the market.

To further complicate matters, some drugs are also classified as:

- **Type AA** — Indicates a drug with potential use for AIDS or HIV- related disease; such drugs are often given a fast-track for potential approval.

- **Type E** — Indicates a drug for a life-threatening or severely debilitating disease; these drugs are also given a priority review and may be used in patients in imminent danger of death.

- **Type F** — Indicates a drug that has been placed on hold until submitted data has been further validated.

- **Type N** — Indicates a drug that is being considered for nonprescription status.

- **Type V** — Indicates a drug that is being considered for "orphan drug" status.

Orphan Drugs

An orphan drug is one that would be difficult for a company to develop into a product because the cost of the NDA process would exceed the anticipated market sales. Usually these drugs are marketed for the treatment of diseases that affect a relatively small patient population.

Rare diseases or conditions are those that affect fewer than 200,000 persons in US. In some cases, orphan drug status may be given to a product that will be useful for more persons if there is no reasonable expectation that cost of development of the product will be recovered by sales of the drug.

The Orphan Drug Act of 1983 encourages companies to develop orphan drugs by giving them incentives such as tax relief, exclusive marketing rights, and faster NDA approval.

Sample Questions

1. How many phases of clinical testing must be conducted before a new drug application may be submitted to the FDA?
   (A) 2   (B) 3   (C) 4   (D) 5   (E) 8

2. The prime purpose of phase 1 clinical trials is to evaluate the drug's
   (A)   therapeutic index
   (B)   safety
   (C)   adverse effects in diseased patients
   (D)   efficacy in diseased patients
   (E)   marketability

3. Phase 1 clinical trials involve subjects that
    (A) are healthy humans without the disease
    (B) lower species of animals
    (C) are primates
    (D) are in a state of disease remission
    (E) have active cases of a disease

4. A clinical pharmacist in a hospital setting is most
    likely to participate in which phase of pre-marketing
    clinical testing?
    (A) 1   (B) 3   (C) 5   (D) 6   (E) 8

5. A pharmaceutical company plans to market a generic
    version of a drug product whose patent has expired.
    Which type of documentation must be submitted to
    the FDA?
    (A) IND   (B) NDA   (C) ANDA
    (D) SNDA   (E) Letter of intent

6. A pharmaceutical company that wishes to lengthen the
    expiration date of a drug product based upon
    additional stability data should submit to the FDA
    a(n):
    (A) IND   (B) NDA   (C) ANDA
    (D) SNDA   (E) Letter of intent

7. Post-marketing surveillance of a new drug product is
    sometimes referred to as the Phase _____ clinical trial.
    (A) 1   (B) 2   (C) 3   (D) 4   (E) 5

8. Which one of the following designations indicates that
    a new drug possesses significant advancement over
    present drug therapy?
    (A) Type 1   (B) Type 2   (C) Type 4
    (D) Type A   (E) Type AB

9. An orphan drug is one that has:
    (A)   been removed from the market because of toxicity
    (B)   been discontinued because of poor sales
    (C)   special economical incentives for the manufacturer
    (D)   a low therapeutic index
    (E)   been developed and imported from a foreign country

10. Some new drug applications are granted a "Type P" status by the FDA. This status implies that the drug
    (A) is for parenteral use
    (B) will be packaged in a novel container
    (C) will receive a low priority (passive) review
    (D) is intended for patients with AIDS (PWA's)
    (E) will receive a priority review of the NDA

Answers: (1) B   (2) B   (3) A   (4) B   (5) C   (6) D
                (7) D   (8) A   (9) C   (10) E

Section E

Requirements for Marketed Drug Products

Naming New Drugs

During the research phases of drug development, the pharmaceutical manufacturer will probably identify an investigational drug by a code name, such as WIN 2306. This avoids the use of the burdensome, long chemical name. Once the drug nears its final approval, a specific name known as the nonproprietary or generic name must be established. The company may also select a trade name or brand name for the drug to encourage prescriber recognition of that company's specific product.

The responsibility for designating a nonproprietary or generic name for a new drug belongs to the United States Adopted Names Council (USAN). This group is sponsored by the American Medical Association (AMA), American Pharmaceutical Association (APhA), and the United States

Pharmacopeial Convention (USPC). However, the Secretary of Human Health Services (HHS) must grant final approval for any drug name. The Secretary may also require the change of a drug name if there appears to be confusion because of two similar drug names (either generic or brand name products).

A distinctive generic name, proprietary name, or USAN is assigned to each new drug based on the following criteria:

- The name should be short, distinctive, and not likely to be confused with other existing names.

- The name should provide some indication of the therapeutic or chemical class to which the drug belongs.

Patent Protection

There are considerable costs and time delays when a company develops a new drug by the submission of an NDA (New Drug Application). In order to allow the company to recover these costs, Congress passed an act to guarantee the innovator company a minimum time period for patent protection before generic versions of the drug product could be marketed.

Up to 1984, innovator companies had a 17-year period of exclusive patent rights, including the development period and the FDA review process. The Drug Price Competition and Patent-Term Restoration Act of 1984, also known as the Waxman-Hatch Amendment, represents a compromise affecting major drug manufacturers and generic companies. The major drug manufacturers were granted longer patent protection (up to an extra five years) while the manufacturers of generic drugs were provided with easier access to approval of their drug applications.

In order to encourage clinical studies of drugs in the pediatric population, the Secretary of HHS may request that such studies be performed if the drug has yet to be approved and may be valuable in pediatrics. An incentive to the pharmaceutical company is an extension of patent protection, usually an additional 6 months. These studies may also be conducted for already marketed drugs and drugs for rare diseases or symptoms.

National Drug Code (NDC)

The NDC is a numbering system that aids in identifying a drug product. Third party payers also employ NDC numbers to identify products for reimbursement.

The NDC of a specific drug product contains ten or eleven digits. For example, a number may be:

1 0 7 4	0 1 2 8	0 4
(manufacturer)	(ID of specific drug)	(ID of package)

Each manufacturer has its own number which has been assigned by the FDA. This number is known as the labeler's code. Each company can then establish its own identification numbers, known as product codes, for a specific drug, its strength, and dosage form. That is, one company might designate warfarin 10mg tablets as 0128 and another company's warfarin 10 mg tablets may be assigned the number 0045. The last two digits usually indicate the package characteristic such as 04 for blister packs or 02 for bottles of 100 tablets.

Newer drug products have either 10 or 11 digit NDC numbers, of which the first five represent the manufacturer and the remaining digits represent the drug and package.

The NDC Directory is a publication that contains listings of NDC numbers and their identity. Other books, such as the Red Book and the Blue Book, as well as the National Drug Code Directory, available at the FDA website, have NDC numbers and their equivalents listed.

All prescription drugs marketed in the United States must have NDC numbers. While placing the NDC number on the package labeling is not mandatory, most companies do so. The NDC number also does not have to appear on individual dosage units nor is there any federal law requiring that NDC numbers appear on prescription labels. However, the NDC serves as a convenient identification tool when transferring information electronically; for example, when requesting reimbursement or ordering drug products.

If a manufacturer discontinues a product, the NDC number may be reassigned to another drug product provided five years has elapsed from the last commercial shipment of the discontinued drug product.

Good Manufacturing Practice (GMP)

Current Good Manufacturing Practice (GMP) is a set of regulations that specify the minimum requirements required to manufacture pharmaceutical products in the US. They are designed to assure safety and quality of pharmaceuticals. Compliance with these regulations is a responsibility of pharmaceutical manufacturers.

While there are many requirements under GMP regulations, this material is unlikely to be tested on the MPJE®. Candidates should, however, be aware that manufacturers must be registered with the FDA and they must describe their manufacturing and production processes as part of the NDA process. The FDA inspects drug manufacturer's facilities approximately once every two years to determine compliance with GMPs, unless a prior history of deficiencies requires more frequent visits.

Adulterated Drug Products

A drug is considered to be adulterated if it:

- contains in whole or in part any filthy, putrid, or decomposed substance.

- has been prepared, packaged, or held under unsanitary conditions where it may have been contaminated.

- has been manufactured under conditions that do not meet the standards of good manufacturing practice (GMPs).

- contains an unapproved color additive.

Product Labeling

The term "label" refers to written, printed, or graphic matter appearing on the immediate container of a drug product. If there is an outside package, any word, statement, or other information present on the immediate container must also appear on the outside package.

The term "labeling" refers to either:

- The information printed on the label and outside package of a drug product. It refers to all labels and other written, printed, or graphic matter either on the product, its container, its wrapper, or accompanying the product. Thus, the prescription drug product insert is considered part of the labeling.

- The information printed by the pharmacist on the prescription label for a drug product being dispensed. (NOTE: The prescription label will be discussed later)

While the original Food, Drug, and Cosmetic Act of 1938 specified that all drug products had to be labeled with "adequate directions for use", the Durham-Humphrey Amendment of 1951 clarified these requirements. It states that drugs do NOT have to have adequate directions for use IF they are intended for dispensing by pharmacists, provided that they contain the legend "Caution: Federal law prohibits dispensing without a prescription". In 1997 this required statement was simplified to read "Rx Only".

Labeling Requirements for Manufacturer's Containers

Federal law requires that the following information appear on manufacturer's containers of drug products:

- Name and address of the manufacturer, packer, or distributor.

- Established name of the drug or drug product.

- The net quantity (weight, quantity, or dosage units) in the package.

- The weight of active ingredient contained in each dosage unit (e.g. 10mg or 2mg/5mL). An additional requirement for electrolyte replacement therapy is inclusion of the electrolyte concentration in terms of milliequivalents (mEq).

- The federal legend "Caution: Federal law prohibits dispensing without a prescription" or the more recent version, "Rx only".

- If dosage units are not taken orally, the specific route or routes of administration must be stated (e.g. for IM or subcutaneous injection).

- Special storage directions, if appropriate.

- Manufacturer's control or lot number.

- The expiration date established by the manufacturer.

If these labeling guidelines are not meticulously adhered to, the product may be considered misbranded. Label errors or omissions that would be considered to be misbranding include:

- A false or misleading label.

- A missing name and location of the manufacturer, packer, or distributor.

- The quantity of the container contents is not present. This could be a numerical count (e.g. 100 tablets), net weight (e.g. 50 g) or net volume (e.g. 4 fl. oz).

- All required information is not prominently displayed so that it can easily be read. This includes the listing of officially designated names of all ingredients.

- Adequate directions for use and appropriate warnings to protect those who use the medication (this applies to nonprescription drugs).

Note

The term "adequate directions for use" in federal laws dealing with OTC labeling means that sufficient information is provided on the labeling so that a layperson could use the product safely.

Listing of Therapeutically Inactive Ingredients on Labels

Inclusion of the names of inactive adjuvants such as antioxidants, buffers, coloring agents, etc. is considered to be good manufacturing practice. All dosage forms must be labeled to state all added ingredients with the exception of flavors and fragrances. Because of the complexity of ingredients in flavoring agents and perfumes, they may be designated by more common names such as cherry flavor or gardenia aroma.

The additives should be listed alphabetically by name but separate from the list of the therapeutically active ingredients. The names should be those used in the official compendia. If not included in these references, the names may be obtained from other sources. The order of preference for these secondary sources is:

- *USP Dictionary of USAN and International Drug Names*
- CTFA *International Cosmetic Ingredient Dictionary and Handbook*
- *Food Chemicals Codex.*

While coloring agents may be present in oral and topical dosage forms, they are expressly prohibited in ophthalmic and parenteral formulations. One type of ingredient found in some parenteral products but not necessarily listed on the label is inert gases that were added for stability purposes.

Package Inserts

Besides the above information, the manufacturer is also required to provide a package insert in prescription drug packages. The information in the package insert must be approved by the FDA and is for informational use only, not for promotional use. The following is required to be included in the package insert:

- Description of the drug (including its solubility, chemical characteristics, etc.)

- Clinical pharmacology

- Indications and usage

- Contraindications

- Warnings

- Precautions

- Adverse reactions

- Potential for abuse or patient dependence

- Symptoms and treatment of overdose

- Dosage and administration

- Available dosage forms of the product

- Date of the most recent revision of the labeling

- Recommended or usual dosage

Identification of Commercial Solid Dosage Forms

The Code of Federal Regulations (CFR) requires manufacturers to imprint solid oral dosage forms, whether they are prescription or nonprescription products. The imprint code must permit the identification of both the manufacturer and the specific drug product. There are some exemptions to this requirement. For example, it is impractical to imprint nitroglycerin sublingual tablets.

Prescription Drug Marketing Act 1987

The Prescription Drug Marketing Act of 1987 (sometimes referred to as the "Dingle bill") was enacted to correct the problem of drug diversion from normal distribution channels. It includes provisions that:

- require proper storage of drugs and the maintenance of appropriate distribution records.

- prohibit companies from shipping drugs between states without being registered in the state from which they are being shipped.

- prohibit drugs from being re-imported into the United States except by the manufacturer of said drugs.

- require state licensing of drug wholesalers.

- restrict the sale, purchase or trade of prescription drug samples and bars retail pharmacies from receiving any prescription drug samples. Drug samples obtained by a practitioner may not be delivered to a retail pharmacy, even if they are to be dispensed to that practitioner's patients. In other words, a retail pharmacy may NOT possess any prescription drug samples obtained from ANY source. Possession of such samples would be considered to be drug diversion by the FDA.

- allows the use of starter packs that contain small quantities of drug product, which are distributed free of charge to pharmacies. They are not considered to be samples since they are intended to be distributed by the pharmacy to initiate drug therapy for a patient. Another mechanism of distributing a drug is by providing vouchers or coupons. The voucher may be filled from pharmacy stock at the manufacturer's expense or at a reduced cost to the patient.

- indicate that hospital or other pharmacies in health care facilities may receive prescription drug samples only if a licensed prescriber has requested them and if precise records are maintained of their disposition. If such samples are received by the pharmacy, they must be stored separately from the normal drug stock.

- prohibit drug products from being resold by hospitals or other health care facilities if they were purchased at special prices. This prevents a hospital pharmacy from purchasing 1000 packages of an antibiotic at a low price then selling a number of them to a community or chain pharmacy in order to make a profit.

- restrict resale of drug products by hospitals or health care facilities.

- permit practitioners licensed to prescribe to receive drug samples provided that a written request is made with their name, address, medical specialty, signature, name of drug, quantity, manufacturer, and date of request. Drug manufacturers and distributors must keep copies of all requests and keep receipts for three years.

- require sales representatives to be responsible for all samples and take an annual inventory.

- establish stiff penalties for violation of this law.

Sample Questions

1. A community pharmacy may fill prescriptions received from a licensed practitioner if based upon receiving a manufacturer's
   I. drug samples
   II. voucher or coupon
   III. starter packs
   (A) I only   (B) III only   (C) I & II only
   (D) II & III only   (E) I, II, & III

2. Commercial oral tablets must have which of the following types of information imprinted on each unit?
   (A)   name of the manufacturer
   (B)   name and strength of the drug
   (C)   a code identifying each of the above
   (D)   the expiration date
   (E)   date of manufacturing

3. Which of the following statements concerning the National Drug Code (NDC) is (are) true?
   I. The NDC must be imprinted on all commercial capsules and tablets.
   II. Only drugs that have an approved new drug application on file may have an NDC.
   III. The NDC may be used for reimbursement purposes.
   (A) I only   (B) III only   (C) I & II only
   (D) II & III only   (E) I, II, & III

4.   A specific drug product has a NDC of 0137-0145-10.
      The 0137 in this designation represents:
      (A) the generic name of the drug
      (B) the location of the company
      (C) the name of the company
      (D) the trade name of the drug
      (E) a unit dose package

5.   Manufacturers will place an NDC on package labels
      for which of the following dosage forms?
      I.   capsules
      II.   oral suspensions
      III. vials of a parenteral solution
      (A) I only   (B) III only   (C) I & II only
      (D) II & III only   (E) I, II, & III

6.   Which of the following commercial products intended
      for oral intake must have identification codes on
      individual dosage units?
      I.   Nonprescription tablet products
      II.   Prescription tablet products
      III. Prescription capsule dosage forms
      (A) I only   (B) III only   (C) I & II only
      (D) II & III only   (E) I, II, & III

Answers: (1)D (2) C (3) B (4) C   (5) E (6) E

Pregnancy Warnings

    Package inserts generally include pregnancy warnings as
part of the "Warnings" section of the insert. Pregnancy
warnings are based on five FDA pregnancy categories.
These include:

- **Category A** - Indicates that there have been adequate, well-controlled studies in pregnant women that demonstrate no risk to the fetus during the first trimester of pregnancy or during the last two trimesters.

- **Category B** - While adequate, well-controlled studies have not been conducted in pregnant women, animal reproduction studies have failed to demonstrate a risk to the fetus.

- **Category C** - The safety of the drug during human pregnancy has not been determined. Animal studies are either positive for fetal risk or have not been conducted. The drug should not be used in human females unless the potential benefit outweighs the potential risk to the fetus.

- **Category D** - There has been positive evidence of risk to the human fetus mainly based upon adverse reaction data from either investigational or marketing experiences. The drug should be administered only if the potential benefits from the use of the drug in pregnant women may be acceptable despite its potential risks.

- **Category X** - Studies in animals, or reports in pregnant women, indicate that the risk of damage caused by the drug clearly outweighs any possible benefit.

Drugs in category X should be considered to be contraindicated in pregnant women or, in most instances, for any woman of childbearing age unless appropriate contraceptive methods are being used. Among the drugs with a Category X rating are Accutane, Cytotec, Thalomid and most "statin" drugs used to reduce serum lipid levels.

The STEPS Program for Thalidomide (Thalomid)

The FDA has established guidelines that a drug company must satisfy in order to distribute a drug that has special safety concerns. Thalidomide is a drug that has historically caused serious teratogenic malformations and was removed from the market in the early 1960's.

Because of new therapeutic indications, Celene has recently reintroduced the drug. This company developed the System for Thalidomide Education and Prescribing Safety (STEPS) to minimize fetal exposure to the drug. Among the elements of this system are:

- Females must undergo pregnancy testing and use effective birth control when being treated with the drug.

- Males must use condoms when having sexual relations.

- All prescribers and pharmacies must be registered in order to prescribe or dispense the drug.

- Use of the drug is monitored by mandatory patient surveys that are sent to a quality assurance committee.

Pharmacies dispensing the drug are limited to prescriptions of up to a 28-day supply with no refills. Written prescriptions must be filled within seven days of being written.

The SMART Program for Isotretinoin (Accutane)

In 2002 Hoffmann-La Roche developed a risk management program with the acronym of SMART (System to Manage Accutane Related Teratogenicity). The program includes requirements for the patient, prescribing physician, and the pharmacist. .

Under this program, a pharmacist may only dispense isotretinoin when a prescription bears a completely and correctly completed yellow self-adhesive label known as the "Accutane Qualification Sticker". One purpose of the Sticker is to assure the pharmacist that the prescriber has determined that his/her patient is qualified to consume this teratogenic drug. By applying this completed sticker, the physician affirms that the patient

- has had two negative pregnancy tests prior to beginning the therapy,
- does not intend to become pregnant during treatment nor for one month after stopping the drug, and,
- is using two forms of birth control simultaneously. It also affirms that the patient has signed an informed consent about the risk of potential birth defects.

Other limitations that the pharmacist must be aware of include the following:

- Not more than a 30 day supply may be dispensed.
- No refills are permitted (a new prescription with the Sticker must be presented for each new supply).

- If the prescription is for a female patient, it must be filled within seven days of the completion of the Sticker.
- All prescriptions for Accutane, including those for males, must bear the Sticker.

Starting in 2004, Roche is packaging all strengths of Accutane in a 30-day supply packaged in six blister packs of ten capsules each. Attached to each blister package are both the Medication Guide (MedGuide) and the Accutane Survey Enrollment Form.

Unapproved Use of Drugs

Can a pharmacist advise a physician regarding the unapproved use or dosage of a drug? Yes! The FDA does not consider prescribing and dispensing drugs for unapproved uses or dosages illegal. Federal law prohibits anyone in the chain of distribution from suggesting to a patient or prescriber that an approved drug may be used for an unapproved purpose. This means that a drug manufacturer cannot promote a drug for a purpose for which it is not indicated. However, the pharmacist may provide drug information about an unapproved use of a drug upon the request of a physician.

In order to study the safety and efficacy of a drug for an unapproved indication, a prescriber should contact the FDA and file a Notice of Claimed Investigational Exemption for a New Drug (IND). The designation, "off-label use", is sometimes used in place of "unapproved use".

Unit-dose packaging and labeling

Many pharmaceutical manufacturers provide their products, especially oral solid dosage forms such as capsules and tablets, in unit-dose packages. These strip packages are convenient for hospital use when daily supplies of the drug for individual patients are sent from the pharmacy to the nursing floors. Because of the small size of these packages, the FDA has issued guidelines as to what information should be on each unit-dose package. This information includes:

- Generic name and trade name, if appropriate.

- Quantity of active drug or drugs present (and number of dosage units if more than one).

- Name of the manufacturer, packer, or distributor.

- The repackager's lot number.

- The expiration date.

- Any other appropriate information concerning the specific drug (e.g. special storage requirements).

Many institutions, especially hospitals, repackage drug products into single dose units. A new expiration date must be provided for the repackaged product since the drug product has been transferred from the manufacturer's container, upon which its original expiration date was provided. Calculations for an appropriate expiration date will be considered later.

The return of unused unit-dose packages to the pharmacy for future dispensing is another issue that must be considered. Most states have established their own regulations. Some allow the return of unit dose packages only if originally dispensed to patients within the hospital setting or in some cases by a community pharmacy to a nursing home.

The expiration-date requirement for a repackaged unit-dose package is fairly strict. While individual state guidelines may vary, the USP/NF states: "in the absence of stability data to the contrary, the expiration date should not exceed 25% of the remaining time between the date of repackaging and the original expiration date OR a six month dating from the date the drug was repackaged, whichever of these two is the LEAST."

Note

The above requirement is stricter than the general requirement in the USP/NF that multiple-unit containers have an expiration date not longer than the expiration date or one year from the date dispensed, whichever is less.

Bar Coding of Pharmaceutical Products

In an attempt to reduce medication errors, the FDA requires pharmaceutical companies to bar code all drug products supplied to hospitals. However, this requirement does not force individual hospitals to utilize bar codes. The ruling applies to prescription, biological, and nonprescription drug products, but not to physician samples. It also applies to single unit containers used in hospital unit-dose drug distribution systems. A bar code consists of a combination of bars and spaces with varying widths that allow encoding of pertinent information concerning a drug product. A scanner is employed in reading the bar code.

Rather than including the drug name, strength or manufacturer, the bar code must contain a drug's NDC. The pharmaceutical manufacturer may include other information that it considers appropriate. While not required, it has been suggested that the drug product's expiration date and lot release number be included.

The Uniform Code Council (UCC) has developed product bar code identification standards for the manufacturing and retail industries. The bar code is considered by the FDA to be a part of the drug product label and is, therefore, subject to good manufacturing practices (GMP). Problems with bar code scanning may be reported to the FDA's Drug Quality Reporting System.

Customized Patient Med Paks

With the consent of the patient, the patient's caregiver, or the prescriber, some pharmacies are providing a customized patient medication package (Med Paks). This package may contain several solid oral dosage forms with directions that specifically indicate the day and time or period of time that the contents of each container are to be taken. The usual information for unit dose packages is required, plus a serial number for the patient Med Pak in addition to the prescription serial numbers for each drug product.

The expiration dating for the Med Pak is based upon the "beyond-use" dating principle but should not exceed 60 days from the date that the Med Pak was prepared.

The MedWatch Program

MedWatch, the FDA Medical Products Reporting Program, is an initiative designed to

- educate all health professionals about the critical importance of being aware of, monitoring for, and reporting adverse events and problems to FDA and/or the manufacturer.

- ensure that new safety information is rapidly communicated to the medical community thereby improving patient care.

The purpose of the MedWatch program is to enhance the effectiveness of post-marketing surveillance of medical products as they are used in clinical practice and to rapidly identify significant health hazards associated with these products.

The MedWatch program has four goals:

- To increase awareness of drug- and device-induced disease

- To clarify what should (and should not) be reported to the agency.

- To make it easier to report problems by operating a single system for health professionals to report adverse events and product problems to the agency.

- To provide regular feedback to the health care community about safety issues involving medical products

Health professionals may report serious adverse events and product problems with all medical products to Med-Watch by mail, phone, fax, or over the Internet. A sample of the MedWatch reporting form is depicted on the following page.

Other Product Reporting Initiatives

Other initiatives exist for health professionals and consumers to report problems with drugs and medical devices. These include the following:

MedMARx™

This system was developed by the USP to allow hospitals to anonymously report, track, and benchmark medication error data. It was developed to help reduce medication errors locally and nationally by permitting users to learn from the adverse experiences of others and share the successful solutions and policies that have been instituted.

Medical Device Problems

Health care facilities (e.g., hospitals, nursing homes, etc.), under the Safe Medical Device Act of 1990 (SMDA), are legally required to report suspected medical device related deaths to both FDA and the manufacturer, if known. Serious injuries must be reported to the manufacturer or to FDA, if the manufacturer is unknown. Health professionals within a health care facility should familiarize themselves with their institution's procedures for SMDA reporting.

U.S. Department of Health and Human Services

Form Approved: OMB No. 0910-0291, Expires: 03/31/03
See OMB statement on reverse.

MedWatch

The FDA Safety Information and
Adverse Event Reporting Program

For VOLUNTARY reporting of
adverse events and product problems

Page _____ of _____

FDA USE ONLY

Triage unit
sequence #

PLEASE TYPE OR USE BLACK INK

A. PATIENT INFORMATION

1. Patient Identifier
In confidence

2. Age at Time of Event:
or
Date of Birth:

3. Sex
☐ Female
☐ Male

4. Weight
lbs
or
kgs

B. ADVERSE EVENT OR PRODUCT PROBLEM

1. ☐ Adverse Event   and/or   ☐ Product Problem (e.g., defects/malfunctions)

2. Outcomes Attributed to Adverse Event (Check all that apply)
☐ Death _____ (mo/day/yr)
☐ Life-threatening
☐ Hospitalization - initial or prolonged
☐ Disability
☐ Congenital Anomaly
☐ Required Intervention to Prevent Permanent Impairment/Damage
☐ Other: _____

3. Date of Event (mo/day/yr)

4. Date of This Report (mo/day/yr)

5. Describe Event or Problem

6. Relevant Tests/Laboratory Data, Including Dates

7. Other Relevant History, Including Preexisting Medical Conditions (e.g., allergies, race, pregnancy, smoking and alcohol use, hepatic/renal dysfunction, etc.)

C. SUSPECT MEDICATION(S)

1. Name (Give labeled strength & manufacturer, if known)
#1
#2

2. Dose, Frequency & Route Used
#1
#2

3. Therapy Dates (If unknown, give duration) from/to (or best estimate)
#1
#2

4. Diagnosis for Use (Indication)
#1
#2

5. Event Abated After Use Stopped or Dose Reduced?
#1 ☐ Yes ☐ No ☐ Doesn't Apply
#2 ☐ Yes ☐ No ☐ Doesn't Apply

6. Lot # (if known)
#1
#2

7. Exp. Date (if known)
#1
#2

8. Event Reappeared After Reintroduction?
#1 ☐ Yes ☐ No ☐ Doesn't Apply
#2 ☐ Yes ☐ No ☐ Doesn't Apply

9. NDC# (For product problems only)

10. Concomitant Medical Products and Therapy Dates (Exclude treatment of event)

D. SUSPECT MEDICAL DEVICE

1. Brand Name

2. Type of Device

3. Manufacturer Name, City and State

4. Model #
Catalog #
Serial #

Lot #
Expiration Date (mo/day/yr)
Other #

5. Operator of Device
☐ Health Professional
☐ Lay User/Patient
☐ Other:

6. If Implanted, Give Date (mo/day/yr)

7. If Explanted, Give Date (mo/day/yr)

8. Is this a Single-use Device that was Reprocessed and Reused on a Patient?
☐ Yes ☐ No

9. If Yes to Item No. 8, Enter Name and Address of Reprocessor

10. Device Available for Evaluation? (Do not send to FDA)
☐ Yes ☐ No ☐ Returned to Manufacturer on _____ (mo/day/yr)

11. Concomitant Medical Products and Therapy Dates (Exclude treatment of event)

E. REPORTER (See confidentiality section on back)

1. Name and Address
Phone #

2. Health Professional?
☐ Yes ☐ No

3. Occupation

4. Also Reported to:
☐ Manufacturer
☐ User Facility
☐ Distributor/Importer

5. If you do NOT want your identity disclosed to the manufacturer, place an "X" in this box: ☐

FDA

Mail to: **MedWatch**
5600 Fishers Lane
Rockville, MD 20852-9787

-or-

FAX to:
1-800-FDA-0178

FORM FDA 3500 (12/03)   Submission of a report does not constitute an admission that medical personnel or the product caused or contributed to the event.

Vaccine Problems

Adverse events and product problems that occur with vaccines should NOT be reported to the MedWatch program or on the MedWatch form but should be sent to the joint FDA/CDC Vaccine Adverse Event Reporting System (VAERS).

Veterinary Product Problems

Adverse events and product problems that occur with the use of medical products (drugs and devices) in animals should be reported to FDA's Center for Veterinary Medicine at 1-888-FDA-VETS (1-888-332-8387).

Drug Recalls

If a marketed drug product exhibits problems, the manufacturer is encouraged to issue a drug recall notice. Problems may vary from minor problems with a particular manufacturing lot to serious drug-related adverse effects such as a high incidence of hepatotoxicity. Drug recalls are divided into three classes.

- **Class I**   The drug product may cause serious, adverse health consequences including death. The recall should include stocks in pharmacies and notification of patients to whom the drug has been dispensed.

- **Class II**   The drug product may cause temporary or reversible effects but the probability of serious adverse effects is remote. The recall will usually include stocks in pharmacies.

- **Class III**   The drug product is unlikely to cause any adverse health consequence.

It is the manufacturer's responsibility to send written recall notices to all wholesalers and pharmacies for recalls in the Class I and II categories. There may be some Class III recalls that are handled with written notices.

It is the pharmacist's responsibility to be aware of all recalls either received in the mail or read in the pharmaceutical literature.

Occasionally, an ingredient present in either a prescription or nonprescription drug product is determined to be potentially dangerous. The FDA may request that a manufacturer of a certain product discontinue sales and/or remove the product from the market. This request for a "voluntary" discontinuation or removal is invariably honored. A recent example of this action was the FDA's request that all companies discontinue marketing products containing phenylpropanolamine(PPA). This was done subsequent to the issuance, by the FDA, of a public health advisory concerning the risk of hemorrhagic stroke or bleeding into the brain linked to the use of PPA.

Prescription Compounding vs. Manufacturing

With the advent of a multitude of commercial prescription drug products, the pharmaceutical industry has relieved the pharmacist of the need for most prescription compounding. The inherent right of the pharmacist to compound prescriptions has been challenged in recent years primarily because of several unfortunate instances in which pharmacists extended their practice into the area of manufacturing.

The critical issue is: When does small-scale prescription compounding become manufacturing? The FDA Compliance Policy Guide of 1992 states that pharmacies may compound drugs extemporaneously if:

- the quantity prepared is reasonable for filling either existing prescriptions or those anticipated based upon prescribing habits of local prescribers and/or prescriptions already on file.

- the dosage forms prepared are not being compounded, provided, or sold to other pharmacies or third-parties such as physician's offices.

- the drug products compounded are not ones already available from commercial sources. That is, they are not compounded versions of FDA-approved drug products.

- the ingredients included in a compounded dosage form meet official standards, usually those found in the USP/NF. If an ingredient does not have an official monograph, it may be used to compound a prescription if it is a component or an approved drug product, or it is on a list of approved substances developed by the Secretary of the U.S. Department of Health and Human Services.

- the pharmacy does not actively solicit business for specific drug products by advertising or by otherwise promoting their compounding capabilities. However, the pharmacy may advertise to both the public and health professionals that it specializes in prescription compounding. The 1997 FDA Modernization Act included a provision that states that compounding pharmacies are not manufacturers and are therefore exempt from standard FDA regulation on that basis. The act prohibited pharmacists from advertising or promoting compounded drugs In 2002, the U.S. Supreme Court modified this policy by ruling that the FDA could not restrict pharmacists from advertising or promoting products solely because they were compounded.

- the pharmacy does not attempt to compound a drug product which is on the list of products that have been withdrawn or removed from the market because they were unsafe or ineffective.

- the pharmacy limits its interstate distribution of compounded products to not more than 5% of the total prescriptions filled by that pharmacy.

May a pharmacist develop a sustained-release drug product similar to a commercial product under his/her prerogative as a compounding pharmacist? The answer is no. This activity is not permissible because a compounding pharmacist is not allowed to compound drug products that are commercially available. In addition, preparing a quantity of the product would probably place the operation into the classification of manufacturing, not compounding.

Expiration Dating for Compounded Prescriptions

The pharmacist should base expiration dating or beyond-use dating upon the stability information available. In the absence of stability information, the following guidelines are appropriate for beyond-use dating.

- For nonaqueous liquids and solids: not more than 25% of the time remaining on the commercial product or a maximum of 6 months, whichever is less.

- For aqueous solutions made from solids obtained from manufactured drug products: 14 days when stored at a cold temperature.

- For all others: the time duration of therapy but not more than 30 days.

Note

Compounded radiopharmaceuticals and positron emission tomography (P.E.T.) drugs are exempt from the compounding standards.

Compounding of Sterile Products for Use in the Home

The USP/NF has issued guidelines for the preparation by pharmacies of sterile drug products intended for dispensing to patients in home settings. These products are designated as "home-use sterile drug products" or "HSD's". The HSD is typically delivered to a residence which is not equipped with a sterile preparation area, and the administration is not under the direct supervision of the dispensing pharmacist.

Such extemporaneously prepared injectable and ophthalmic drug products must be compounded in a strictly-defined environment to assure sterility and safety. Techniques required to prepare such products are classified as "low–risk" or "high-risk" mainly based upon the types of ingredients to be used, dosage forms to be prepared, and the aseptic techniques required.

Low-Risk

These are techniques involving commercially available sterile products that are manufactured in a "closed system". Examples include:

- transfer of a solution from a commercial vial or ampule with a needle and syringe

- compounding total parenteral nutrition (TPN) solutions using commercially available sterile solutions

- transfer of sterile solutions into elastomeric devices

High Risk

These are techniques involving more complex skills to assure sterility and safety of the final product. Such techniques are further categorized as Category I or Category II.

Category I activities include the following techniques:

- pooling sterile drug products for subsequent transfers

- complex compounding involving numerous aseptic processes

- preparing an infusion intended for multi-day use in a portable pump or reservoir system

An example of a Category I compounding activity would be the preparation of TPN's using automated compounding devices.

Category II activities involve ingredients, products, and techniques which pose the greatest risk of contamination. In most instances, the final product will have to be sterilized by the compounder. Examples would include:

- using non-sterile drug substances in the preparation of a product

- using "open systems" such as the compounding of morphine solutions for injection or infusion using morphine powder

- compounding sterile nutritional solutions using non-sterile ingredients during which the initial mixing is performed in an unsealed or nonsterile reservoir.

Sample Questions

1. Which of the following actions is (are) permissible under the FDA rules for prescription compounding by pharmacies?
   I.   Advertising to eye doctors that the pharmacy can compound sterile, isotonic ophthalmic solutions.
   II. Sending brochures to nurse practitioners that indicate that the pharmacy compounds topical ointments for the treatment of skin rashes.
   III. Informing an allergy specialist that the pharmacy can economically compound 50 mg diphenhydramine capsules.
   (A) I only   (B) III only   (C) I & II only
   (D) II & III only   (E) I, II, & III

2. A pharmacy begins to receive prescriptions for a capsule mixture that is not available commercially. The usual prescription is for 14 capsules to be taken once a day with two refills. What is the maximum number of capsules the pharmacist may compound under FDA guidelines?
   (A)   14 only
   (B)   28 only
   (C)   42 only
   (D)   not more than 100
   (E)   a sufficient quantity to meet anticipated prescriptions and refills

3. Which of the following actions may a pharmacy that is specializing in extemporaneous compounding undertake?
   I.   advertise and promote with a brochure its compounding services
   II.   describe its capabilities to prepare sterile parenteral admixtures
   III.   describe dollar savings to customers of a compounded pilocarpine 2% ophthalmic solution
   (A) I only   (B) III only   (C) I & II only
   (D) II & III only   (E) I, II, & III

4. A pharmaceutical manufacturer includes a color additive, that is not FDA approved, in a topical cream formulation. The product could be removed from the market as being:
   (A) adulterated   (B) contaminated
   (C) improperly labeled   (D) misbranded
   (E) hyperallergenic

5. The number of categories of drug recalls is __?__ with recall number __?__ the most serious.
   (A) 3 and 1   (B) 3 and 3   (C) 4 and 1
   (D) 4 and 4   (E) 5 and 1

6. Which of the following techniques would be classified as "low-risk" for pharmacists to perform based upon USP guidelines for preparation of home-use sterile drug products?

   I.   Placing 20 mEq of Potassium Chloride Injection into a 1 liter bag of Sterile D/W using a needle and syringe
   II. Mixing 500 mL of a Sterile Amino Acids Solution with 500 mL of D50W by gravity flow.
   III. Aseptically transferring 20 mL of sterile Morphine Sulfate Injection into a 50 mL elastomeric device.

   (A) I only   (B) III only   (C) I & II only
   (D) II & III only (E) I, II, & III

7. Which of the following techniques would be classified as "high-risk, Category II" for pharmacists to perform based upon USP guidelines for preparation of home-use sterile drug products?
   I.   Compounding an injection solution using nonsterile drug powder and then passing the solution through a 0.22 micron filter.
   II. Mixing several sterile solutions together to make a batch of TPN injections.
   III. Pooling several vials of a chemotherapeutic drug injection for subsequent subdivision into individual minibags.

   (A) I only   (B) III only   (C) I & II only
   (D) II & III only   (E) I, II, & III

Answers: (1) C   (2) E   (3) C   (4) A
          (5) A   (6) E   (7) A

Section F

Filling and Dispensing Prescriptions

Whenever the pharmacist encounters a prescription or medication order for a specific drug product, one of his/her first considerations should be whether the drug is classified as a non-controlled prescription drug or as a controlled substance. Most controlled substance regulations are stricter than those for other drug products, particularly with respect to inventory requirements, limits on quantities that may be dispensed and labeling requirements.

Controlled substance regulations will be covered in great detail in Section G of this Guide. In this section the general regulations for the filling and dispensing of prescriptions will be considered, i.e. rules that apply to almost all prescription products.

Federal vs. State Regulations

Federal and individual state pharmacy laws sometimes differ. In these instances, the more strict regulation usually predominates and must be followed.

> ## Note
> The individuals responsible for the MPJE® are careful to avoid questions that fall into the "gray area" i.e., those questions concerning areas of pharmacy practice which either have conflicting regulations between the federal and state governments or involve issues that have not been clearly resolved. For example, there may be court cases that have not yet been decided regarding conflicting laws. Before a question is accepted as a test item, its worthiness is evaluated by being tested as a sample question on other examinations. As explained previously, always choose the stricter law or regulation when there is a conflict between federal law and state law. The following guidelines may be helpful when answering MPJE® questions.

Authorization to Prescribe

Each state specifies those types of health professionals who may prescribe and set limits of prescribing on prescribers such as nurse practitioners, physician assistants, etc. Questions in this area are usually based on individual state laws.

Health Professionals That Self-prescribe

Can a legitimate prescriber write a prescription for his/her own use? Self-prescribing is acceptable in most states, but some have prohibited the self-prescribing of controlled substances.

Pharmacist's Obligation to Fill a Prescription

A pharmacist may refuse to fill any prescription for any one of several "good" reasons including:

- The prescription is a suspected forgery or fictitious. The difference between these two terms is mainly one of semantics. A forged prescription is one which has been written using the name and information of a legitimate prescriber. A fictitious prescription is one which someone has prepared by creating information based upon a nonexistent prescriber.

- The pharmacist will be violating the law if he/she fills the prescription.

- The drug or drug product is not in stock.

- The pharmacist believes that the drug product may be harmful to the patient.

Prescription Refills

One issue that faces every prescriber and dispenser is whether a specific prescription may be refilled. Controlled substances have tighter limitations as to whether or how often a prescription may be refilled. To refill a prescription for other drugs, the prescriber must have indicated how many refills he/she wishes the patient to have and/or a time limitation for refills to be obtained. Many states have established stricter limitations, usually a time span of not more than one year. All refills must be indicated on the back of the original prescription or by using another reliable system (e.g. a computer).

If a pharmacist receives a prescription for a nonprescription drug product with specific refill directions he/she is bound to the refill limits, particularly if the dose prescribed is greater than normal or if the drug is a Schedule V controlled substance.

Prescription Ownership

Once a prescription has been filled and dispensed, the prescription is legally owned by the pharmacy. It should not be removed from the files except by court order. If the prescriber or patient requests the actual prescription, the pharmacist should refuse but offer a copy of the prescription.

Prescription File Storage Period

Once a prescription has been dispensed, the federal or state law requires pharmacists to maintain the original prescription on file for at least 3 to 5 years.

Labeling of Prescription Drugs

The nature of information that must be on a prescription label depends upon whether the drug is a controlled substance or non-controlled. It also depends on whether an individual state has requirements more stringent than federal guidelines. The FDCA requires that every prescription must be labeled with:

- Name of the patient
- Prescription (serial) number
- Date when the prescription is either written or dispensed (some states require that the date of a refill be used when a prescription is refilled.)
- Directions for use of the drug product by the patient
- Name of the prescriber
- Name and address of the pharmacy
- Any special cautionary statements that may be appropriate.

Note that the above minimum requirements do not mention expiration dating, lot number of the drug product, name of the drug, manufacturer, or strength. This type of information, although valuable, is not required by federal law and is left to the discretion of the individual states.

Expiration Dating vs. Beyond Use Dating

While the term "expiration date" originated with the dating required on manufacturer's containers, the term "beyond-use date" is now used to describe the dating of drug products that are dispensed by pharmacists. The simplest example would be an antibiotic powder, which is reconstituted with purified water by the pharmacist. The traditional "beyond-use" expiration date for the reconstituted antibiotic solution is typically ten days, even though the "expiration date" indicated on the manufacturer's container may be two years for the unreconstituted powder.

The USP has issued guidelines for dispensing pharmacists with regard to beyond-use dating. For oral solid dosage forms, the beyond-use date is somewhat arbitrary depending upon the pharmacist's professional judgment or specific state regulations. In all cases, the beyond-use date may not be greater than the expiration date on the manufacturer's original package. For other dosage forms in multi-dose containers, the beyond-use date must be the shorter of either the manufacturer's expiration date or not more than one year from the date the drug is dispensed.

While regulations dealing with expiration dates for drug products dispensed by prescription are in the hands of the individual states, the FDA specifies that labels for drug products dispensed to nursing homes, intermediate care, and skilled nursing facilities must have beyond-use dating.

Questions concerning expiration dating must be answered carefully since there are several possible scenarios that involve expiration dating. These include:

- **Expiration dating for a commercial drug product as established by the manufacturer.**
  The manufacturer has established this dating for a specific package and a specific product. Most manufacturers indicate the expiration date on the container in terms of month and year. For example, the designation of July 2007 indicates that the manufacturer has data showing that the drug product will remain within USP/NF specifications at least through July 31, 2007. Homeopathic products are exempted from the requirement of an expiration dating.

- **Expiration dating for a unit dose package that has been prepared from a bulk container of a commercial drug product.**
  The re-packager, usually a pharmacist who is supervising the operation, will determine this dating. The current guideline provided in the USP/NF is for re-

packaged drug products to have the shorter of two potential dates:

- 6 months maximum or

- 25% of the time remaining on the original package of bulk drug product.

Many states, however, have established other guidelines by allowing longer dating - as much as one year maximum or 50% of the time remaining on the manufacturer's expiration date, whichever is less. Since the USP is presently reviewing its guidelines, it is unlikely that the MPJE® will have questions on expiration dating for unit-dose packages.

Study Tip

One possible question that could be asked is how the FDA and other inspection bodies classify a unit dose product that does not have an expiration date? The answer is that the product is assumed to be misbranded.

Sample Calculation

Assume that an original drug product had an expiration date of Sept 2006. A pharmacist repackages the product on January 1, 2006 and uses the FDA guidelines of six months maximum or 25% of the time remaining on the original package of bulk drug product.

A six-month maximum will produce a useful product life of January through June and will result in the expiration date of June 2006. The rule using 25% of time remaining will result in the calculation of 25% of the time from the date of repackaging to the manufacturer's expiration date (a total period of nine months). Twenty-five percent of nine months is 2.25 months, thereby yielding the expiration date of March 7, 2006.

In the above example the March date is shorter than the June date and must be used. Be careful! An answer of March 2006 would be incorrect since that implies an expiration date of March 31, 2006. If the choices of answers are (A) Jan 2006 (B) Feb 2006 (C) Mar 2006 (D) June 2006 (E) Sept 2006, you would have to select (B) as the correct choice. Hopefully the examiners will not be this tricky!

- **Expiration dating for individual prescriptions being dispensed by a pharmacist.**
    There is no federal law concerning this type of dating. Instead, some states have established their own guidelines, usually a maximum of one year.

- **Manufacturer's expiration dating.**
    All pharmaceuticals must have a clearly legible expiration date on the package. The manufacturer establishes the expiration date for a commercial drug product by conducting extensive stability testing of the drug dosage form in the final package. Data is submitted to the FDA to validate the dating, which is usually a time span of several years.
    Most manufacturers indicate the expiration date on the container labeling in terms of month and year. For example, the designation of July 2006 indicates that the manufacturer has data showing that the drug product will remain within USP/NF specifications at least through July 31, 2006. To be more specific, if the official standards for a 100 mg tablet is "not less than 95% of labeled claim", one would expect that on July 31st,

the active amount of drug in the tablet would not be less than 95 mg.

Pharmacists may not continue to dispense a drug product once its expiration date has passed. Most states require the pharmacist to remove any expired products from the working stock to an isolated area until the product can either be destroyed or returned to the manufacturer.

Poison Prevention Packaging Act (PPPA)

The purpose of the Poison Prevention Packaging Act (PPPA) of 1970 is to provide special packaging to protect children under the age of five years of age from accidental poisoning. Almost all prescription drugs, nonprescription drugs, and household products must have safety closures that prevent access to young children.

Included in these provisions are the following:

- If an OTC product is marketed in several sizes, one package size is not required to have a safety closure. Such products must include on their label a statement, "This package for households without young children."

- All new and refilled prescriptions must be dispensed in a child-resistant closure unless:

  - the prescriber specifies that none is to be used. This may only be specified for cach individual prescription, i.e. a physician cannot provide a blanket child-resistant waiver directive.

  - the patient indicates that they do not want such a closure. Patients may ask for a non-child-resistant container for a single prescription or they may pro-vide a "blanket waiver" that directs the pharmacist to never provide a child-resistant container. In either case, it is advisable to have the patient sign a waiver on the back of each individual prescription and to reconfirm the patient's wishes on a regular basis.

- the container is being used in a hospital or similar institution in which the drugs are maintained and administered by health professionals. However, child-resistant containers should be used by phar-macies providing drug products to nursing homes.

Note

Pharmacists may not use a single patient request for a non-child-resistant container as justification to dispense future prescriptions in such containers.

- When preparing prescription refills for patients, both parts (body and closure) of plastic container units must be replaced. If the container body is constructed of glass, it may be reused but the plastic closure must be replaced. This is a safety precaution since many plastic closures may lose their child-resistant features after re-peated use. The pharmacy may employ reversible closures (those de-signed to be used as either safety or regular tops) although this practice is discouraged by the CPSC.

Some drug products are exempt from the PPPA by special request of the manufacturer. Examples include:

- Sublingual nitroglycerin tablets.

- Sublingual and chewable isosorbide dinitrate products in doses of 10 mg or less.

- Aspirin and acetaminophen effervescent tablets or granules.

- Oral contraceptives in memory-aid packages (e.g. dial-packs). These packages, which assist the patient's memory, are known as mnemonic packages and usually allow the dispensing of tablets one at a time.

- Potassium supplements in unit dose packaging.

- Sodium fluoride products containing not more than 264 mg of sodium fluoride per package.

- Anhydrous cholestyramine and colestipol packets.

- Products in aerosol containers intended for inhalation therapy.

Note

Recent additions to the PPPA include regulations about iron-containing products. These include:

- Products containing 30 mg of elemental iron or more must be packaged in unit dose containers.

- Packages that contain more than 250 mg of elemental iron must be child-resistant.

Some drug products are intended by the pharmaceutical manufacturer to be dispensed in their original containers by the pharmacist. Such units must also meet the requirements of the Poison Prevention Packaging Act (PPPA).

The Consumer Product Safety Commission (CPSC), which has jurisdiction of the PPPA, has revised the testing protocols for child-resistant packaging (CRP). Test panels used to assess such packaging will consist of two groups:

- Children under five years of age.
- Adults 50 to 70 years of age.

This replaces the requirement for an adult panel that was comprised of 18 to 45 year old adults. A package will fail the child-resistant test if more than 20% of the children can open the package in a total of ten minutes. However, to meet adult-friendly requirements, 90% of a one hundred person adult panel must be able to open and close the package in five minutes; and then do so a second time within one minute.

Federal Anti-Tampering Act (1982)

Following several incidents of deliberate contamination of OTC products with poisonous substances, Congress enacted the Federal Anti-Tampering Act in 1982. Provisions of this Act require that tamper-evident packaging be used for select OTC products and cosmetics, particularly those taken orally. The package may feature an indicator or barrier to limit access. If disturbed, some visible evidence of entry will be evident. For example, a simple plastic film seal or a tab around the container closure is sufficient. The product label must indicate that it is a tamper-evident package and should indicate how a consumer can determine if the package has been tampered with.

> ## Note
> In reviewing this chapter, remember that the tamper-evident and the poison prevention regulations are different.

Sample Questions

1. Enforcement of the PPPA is basically under the jurisdiction of the:
   (A)   Consumer Product Safety Commission (CPSC)
   (B)   Federal Trade Commission (FTC)
   (C)   Food and Drug Administration (FDA)
   (D)   Federal Alcohol, Tobacco and Firearms Agency
   (E)   Health Care Financing Administration (HCFA)

2. Permission to not use a poison prevention closure on a prescription may be granted by the
   I.   patient
   II.   prescriber
   III.   pharmacist
   (A) I only   (B) III only   (C) I & II only
   (D) II & III only   (E) I, II, & III

3. The Poison Prevention Packaging Act (PPPA) was intended to protect
   I.   visually impaired patients
   II.   geriatric patients
   III.   young children
   (A) I only   (B) III only   (C) I & II only
   (D) II & III only   (E) I, II, & III

4. When refilling a prescription that requires a poison pre-
   vention container, the pharmacist must always replace
   a
   I.   glass container
   II.   plastic container
   III. plastic closure
   (A) I only   (B) III only   (C) I & II only
   (D) II & III only   (E) I, II, & III

5. Original packages of nitroglycerin, which are exempt
   from the requirements of the Poison Prevention
   Packaging Act, include:
   I.   sublingual tablets
   II.   ointments
   III. oral tablets
   (A) I only   (B) III only   (C) I & II only
   (D) II & III only   (E) I, II, & III

6. In which of the following situations are child-resistant
   closures not required?
   I.   When a prescriber dispenses a prescription drug
        directly from his/her office.
   II. When a hospital pharmacy fills a prescription
        for an outpatient.
   III. When a hospital pharmacy fills a prescription for
        an inpatient.
   (A) I only   (B) III only   (C) I & II only
   (D) II & III only   (E) I, II, & III

7. Which of the following types of drug products are not
   required to be dispensed in a poison prevention
   package?

    (A)   An analgesic for a child over the age of two
    (B)   An analgesic for a child over the age of five
    (C)   An analgesic for an adult
    (D)   A bronchodilator in a metered aerosol container
    (E)   Estrogen tablets for a female over the age of 65

8.   Which of the following OTC products must be packaged in a tamper-evident package?
    I.   mouthwash
    II.   contact lens solution
    III.   insulin
    (A) I only   (B) III only   (C) I & II only
    (D) II & III only   (E) I, II, & III

Answers: (1) A   (2) C   (3) B   (4) D   (5) C   (6) B
              (7) D   (8) C

Patient Package Inserts (PPIs)

Many potentially dangerous drugs must be dispensed with a Patient Package Insert (PPI). This is a document, written in lay language, that is intended to educate the client about the proper use and potential dangers inherent in the use of the product accompanying the PPI. PPIs must be provided to patients receiving prescriptions for products such as Accutane, HMG-CoA reductase inhibitors (i.e. the "statin" drugs), as well as those receiving estrogen or pro-gesterone-containing products. Patients receiving these drugs must receive a PPI prior to administration of the first dose of the medication and every 30 days thereafter as long as the therapy continues.

These rules apply to all physicians, community pharm-acists, and hospital pharmacists who dispense the drugs. It also means that hospital pharmacies must provide patient package inserts to hospitalized patients who are receiving estrogen and progestin-containing products such as Premarin, oral contraceptive products, and intrauterine contraceptive devices containing these drugs. This may be done by providing patients with the PPI prior to administering the first dose of such drug products and once every thirty days thereafter. This PPI requirement also applies to patients in long term care facilities such as nursing homes.

Prescribers who dispense prescriptions from their offices are NOT exempt from the requirement of providing PPIs.

Medication Guides

As part of an initiative to provide patients with comprehensive information about drug products that have been prescribed for them, the FDA, in 1995, announced the Medication Guide program. This program provides standards for the distribution and quality of written prescription information material or Medication Guides to be dispensed to patients. Such guides would be prepared by drug manufacturers on a voluntary basis and in language easily understood by patients. The Guides would be provided to dispensers, who would be required to provide them to patients.

Drug Product Substitution

The regulations that describe the process of substitution of one drug product for another are within the jurisdiction of individual states. Candidates should carefully review the mechanisms and limitations of substitution for pharmacists in the state(s) in which they are attempting to be licensed.

The premise of simple substitution is to provide a lower cost drug product in place of the drug product prescribed. A key factor in substitution has been the necessity that the originally prescribed drug and the substituted drug products had to be PHARMACEUTICALLY equivalent. That is, each drug product must have the same active ingredient, same dosage form, same route of administration, and be identical in strength or concentration. Pharmaceutically equivalent products may, however, contain different excipients.

The term, THERAPEUTIC equivalence is used to denote drug products that are
- pharmaceutical equivalents AND
- bioequivalent.

Drug products that are considered to be bioequivalent have been clinically evaluated and have been shown to have similar pharmacokinetic properties. That is, a similar ADME pathway. ADME is the acronym for
- Absorption
- Distribution
- Metabolism
- Elimination

Data submitted to the FDA by a manufacturer will include graphs that illustrate that two products containing the same drug have similar blood concentration versus time curves. Most critical in claiming bioequivalence is that two products each produce similar
- time to peak
- peak concentrations
- area under the curve (AUC)

The FDA will generally approve the marketing of competing drug products if they are shown not to present bioequivalence problems or, if they do present a potential problem, they are shown to meet appropriate bioequivalence standards.

A third designation, "pharmaceutical alternatives", refers to drug products that contain the same therapeutic moiety BUT may consist of different

- salts
- esters or complexes
- dosage forms
- strengths

Most states do not allow substitution between pharmaceutical alternatives, so they will not be considered in this Guide.

While simple drug substitution is self-explanatory, the term "therapeutic substitution" is more complex. This term is used when a pharmacy has the right to substitute a different drug for the one designated on the prescription or medical order, without contacting the prescriber (e.g. one cephalosporin drug for another). This practice is generally limited to institutions that utilize a drug formulary.

A committee within the institution (usually the Pharmacy and Therapeutics Committee) generally determines which drug products will be included in the formulary. All participating prescribers agree to abide by the approved therapeutic substitution policies. The intent of the drug formulary is to save the institution money by utilizing more economical drug products in a certain therapeutic area and also by reducing the need for the institution to maintain a large drug inventory.

The term "closed formulary" refers to a formulary where only the drug products listed may be used, while the term "open formulary" is used to describe a formulary that permits some unlisted drug products to be dispensed.

When the prescriber writes or the pharmacist selects a drug product for dispensing, one of the following three types of drug names may be used:

- **Generic name** - This is the single specific name given to a drug by the USAN. In the United States each specific drug structure is given only one generic name. For example, ampicillin denotes a chemical that has a specific chemical structure.

- **Trade name or Brand name** - This unique name is selected by a pharmaceutical company for its own brand of a generic drug. For example, Apothecon has selected Polycillin as a trade name for their brand of ampicillin while GlaxoSmithKline has registered the trade name of Totacillin. The purpose of a brand name is to encourage prescribers to prescribe a specific company's product exclusively. Remember that every drug product that has been given a trade name or a brand name still has the same, original generic name as every other drug product containing the same active ingredient.

Some prescribers will write both the generic name and the manufacturer's name on a prescription (e.g. ampicillin-Premium Labs). When this occurs, the pharmacist must realize that this is equivalent to writing either a trade name or brand name. In this example, the pharmacist is obligated to dispense Premium Lab's ampicillin product.

A new drug product will often have patent protection for a number of years. Its manufacturer has exclusive rights for marketing the drug product and has likely chosen a trade name for the product. The drug product may be referred to as a "Single Source Product" since no other manufacturer markets the same drug. Once the patent has expired, other companies may submit ANDAs to gain approval for their marketing of the same drug. They may choose to use only the generic name or they may select their own exclusive brand name. When more than one manufacturer has a drug product on the market, the term "Multisource Product" is used.

Since pharmacokinetic data for new drug products are sent to the FDA for review, it is logical that the FDA will supply health professionals with bioequivalence information. A publication containing this information is known as *Approved Drug Products with Therapeutic Equivalence Evaluations*, better known as the "*The Orange Book*". Monthly supplements are issued for *The Orange Book*. An electronic version of *The Orange Book* is also available. There are several other reference sources available for determining the status of a specific drug product. These include:

- *United States Pharmacopeia Dispensing Information (USP/DI) Volume III* plus supplements

- *Facts and Comparisons, Inc. Approved Bioequivalence Codes*

- FDA's Internet Web site: http://www.fda.gov

Whenever an innovator's new drug product is developed and submitted with a New Drug Application (NDA), it becomes the reference standard. Manufacturers interested in marketing a product that attempts to duplicate the innovator's drug product must submit to the FDA an Abbreviated New Drug Application (ANDA).

The bioequivalence of the generic versions of an innovator's drug product must be determined. Based on such testing, generic products are classified in one of two categories:

- **"A" rated products** - Such products are determined to be bioequivalent and are thus "therapeutically equivalent" to the brand name or reference product.

- **"B" rated products** - These are products that are found not to be bioequivalent.

Products that are A-rated may be substituted for one another while B-rated products cannot. Most states, however, limit substitution to interchanges between products that are the same dosage form. That is, one cannot substitute a capsule dosage form with a tablet dosage form or an ointment for a cream. Also, most sustained-release or controlled-release dosage forms are not interchangeable.

To further clarify the meaning of these codes, products assigned the "A" code are generally placed into one of several subcategories that generally designate different dosage forms. These subcategories include:

- **AA**   Drug products in conventional dosage forms

- **AN**   Solutions and powders for aerosolization

- **AO**   Injectable products with oil solvents

- **AP**   Injectable solutions

- **AT**   Topical products (if they are the same dosage form)

<hr>

Study Tip

It is probably not necessary to learn these subcategories.

<hr>

Some drug products identified by the FDA as having actual or potential bioequivalence problems may be acceptable substitutes if the equivalency problem has been resolved by *in vivo* and/or *in vitro* studies. Such drug products are given an "AB" designation, which signifies that the product meets "necessary bioequivalence requirements".

To summarize, products with similar "A" codes and having the same dosage strength may be substituted for each other while products with "B" codes cannot.

The FDA has further expanded this code system by designating some AB products as AB1, AB2, AB3, etc. These subcategories are intended to categorize drug products, which previously would not be considered bioequivalent into bioequivalent groups. The best examples of the use of these subcategories are the transdermal nitroglycerin patches. Originally these were classified as "B" since their release mechanisms varied from product to product. However, they are now classified as follows:

Product	Category
NitroDur transdermal (Key) (the reference standard)	AB1
Minitran Transdermal (3M)	AB1

Product	Category
Transderm-Nitro (Summit) (the reference standard)	AB2
NTG transdermal (Mylan)	AB2

Thus NitroDur and Minitran transdermal systems are considered bioequivalent to each other and the Transderm-Nitro and NTG transdermal systems (Mylan) are considered bioequivalent to one another. However, one cannot substitute Transderm-Nitro for NitroDur, or Minitran for Transderm-Nitro.

Another group of drug products with fairly lenient substitution regulations is the amino acid solutions used for preparing TPN's. These are classified as exceptions to the bioequivalence regulations. Such solutions may vary slightly in composition from one another, but it is unlikely that there would be significant differences in therapeutic activity between them as long as the total percentage of amino acids is the same in each. The pharmacist is permitted to substitute such amino acids solutions relatively freely.

As mentioned previously, the "B" codes are assigned to drug products that the FDA does not currently consider to be therapeutically equivalent to other pharmaceutically equivalent products. Since bioequivalence problems often stem from dosage form problems, codes of BC, BD, BE, BP, BR, BS, BT, BX, and B* are sometimes assigned to such products. The meaning of these is listed below:

- **BC**   Extended-release dosage forms (capsules, tablets, injectables)

- **BD**   Active ingredients and dosage forms with documented bioequivalence problems

- **BE**   Delayed-release oral dosage forms (e.g. enteric coated tablets)

- **BN**   Aerosol-nebulizer drug delivery systems

Note

Metered aerosol dosage forms are not to be considered bioequivalent unless the drug products meet an appropriate bioequivalence standard.

- **BP**   Active ingredients and dosage forms with potential bioequivalence problems.
  (e.g. injectable suspensions)

- **BR**   Suppositories or enemas that are intended for systemic absorption

- **BS**   Products that have drug standard deficiencies (e.g. a drug that contains several active components.

- **BT**   Topical products with bioequivalence issues

- **BX**   Drug products with insufficient data to determine therapeutic equivalence;
also used to denote a drug product likely to lose its FDA approval

---

Study Tip

Good news! It is unlikely that any question will be asked where you must know the difference between any of the above "B" categories.

What is the status of a drug that is manufactured by the New Drug Application holder (i.e. the innovator) but is being repackaged and/or distributed by another company? Since the original company holding the NDA manufactures it, the product meets all bioequivalence requirements and will thus be considered bioequivalent.

Some drugs and their related drug products marketed before 1938 are not required to be listed in the Orange Book because they have a "Grandfather" exemption. Included in this category are drugs such as ASA with codeine, codeine, digoxin, ephedrine, epinephrine, levothyroxine, morphine, nitroglycerin, phenobarbital, oral potassium chloride preparations, pseudoephedrine, thyroid, and quinine.

In addition, some generic forms of nitroglycerin transdermal systems marketed prior to 1962 are exempt as well. While many of these products had bioavailability data, they did not have appropriate bioequivalence data. Over the past few years, however, many of these multi-source products have been listed in the Orange Book because their manufacturers recognize the value of providing substitution information.

Narrow Therapeutic Index Drugs (NTI's)

The term, Narrow Therapeutic Index or Narrow Therapeutic Ratio refers to drugs where the multiple between the minimum toxic concentration and the minimum effective concentration is relatively low (i.e. two or less). Examples of such drugs include digoxin, levothyroxine, lithium, phenytoin, theophylline, valproic acid and warfarin. A few states, but not the federal government, have passed their own regulations limiting the free substitution of different manufacturers' products.

Using the Orange Book

The Orange Book is available in two formats, in hard copy or as the Electronic Orange Book at the FDA Internet website (http://www.fda.gov/cder/ob/default.htm).   Each source provides interested parties with the opportunity to find and compare therapeutic equivalence (TE) codes for multi-source products. The bound edition of the Orange Book is published each year and is regularly updated during each year. The Electronic Orange Book is updated continuously.

Tables I-IV are abridged sections taken from the electronic version of The Orange Book current in Fall, 2004. The left hand column on these tables lists the Therapeutic Equivalence Evaluations (TE) Bioequivalence Code This is important information for the pharmacist because it indicates the bioequivalence status of each drug product. The second column from the left indicates whether the product is a Reference Listed Drug (RLD) or not.   RLD drugs are generally the innovator drugs that represent the standard used by new applicants to apply for an ANDA.

Tables I and II present information about the tablet forms of the drug verapamil HCl (a generic name). Note that various dosage strengths are listed with their corresponding manufacturers. If a specific manufacturer uses a trade name or brand name, the drug product is listed by that name. Otherwise, just the generic name is listed. Note that the first oral tablet of verapamil HCl listed is

Abbott's Isoptin in 40, 80, and 120 mg strengths, all rated AB. The next product is GD Searle's Calan in 40, 80, and 120 mg strengths also rated AB. Therefore, substitution among these two bioequivalent TABLET products is possible provided the same dosage strength is used.

Note that the 120 mg Isoptin Oral Tablet product (the only product with a "Yes" in the RLD column) was the reference standard used by the FDA for bioequivalence comparisons.

Next, verapamil hydrochloride tablets manufactured by four different companies are listed. All of these have AB ratings and are, therefore, interchangeable with either Calan or Isoptin.

Table II depicts an abridged version of the Electronic Orange Book listing for extended-release verapamil tablet products. Note that Covera-HS is the reference standard used by the FDA for bioequivalence study comparisons. Also note that this product, manufactured by GD Searle LLC, has a status of BC, indicting a lack of bioequivalence. In this case, bioequivalence problems are likely when comparing this product with the action of other extended-release verapamil products because of the special release system for the product.

TE Code	RLD	Active Ingredient	Dosage Form; Route	Strength	Proprietary Name	Applic
AB	Yes	VERAPAMIL HYDROCHLORIDE	Tablet; Oral	120MG	ISOPTIN	ABBOTT
AB	No	VERAPAMIL HYDROCHLORIDE	Tablet; Oral	40MG	ISOPTIN	ABBOTT
AB	No	VERAPAMIL HYDROCHLORIDE	Tablet; Oral	80MG	ISOPTIN	ABBOTT
AB	No	VERAPAMIL HYDROCHLORIDE	Tablet; Oral	120MG	CALAN	GD SEAR LLC
AB	No	VERAPAMIL HYDROCHLORIDE	Tablet; Oral	40MG	CALAN	GD SEAR LLC
AB	No	VERAPAMIL HYDROCHLORIDE	Tablet; Oral	80MG	CALAN	GD SEAR LLC
AB	No	VERAPAMIL HYDROCHLORIDE	Tablet; Oral	120MG	VERAPAMIL HCL	SANDOZ
AB	No	VERAPAMIL HYDROCHLORIDE	Tablet; Oral	40MG	VERAPAMIL HCL	SANDOZ
AB	No	VERAPAMIL HYDROCHLORIDE	Tablet; Oral	80MG	VERAPAMIL HCL	SANDOZ
AB	No	VERAPAMIL HYDROCHLORIDE	Tablet; Oral	120MG	VERAPAMIL HCL	PUREPAC
AB	No	VERAPAMIL HYDROCHLORIDE	Tablet; Oral	80MG	VERAPAMIL HCL	PUREPAC
AB	No	VERAPAMIL HYDROCHLORIDE	Tablet; Oral	120MG	VERAPAMIL HCL	PLIVA
AB	No	VERAPAMIL HYDROCHLORIDE	Tablet; Oral	40MG	VERAPAMIL HCL	PLIVA
AB	No	VERAPAMIL HYDROCHLORIDE	Tablet; Oral	80MG	VERAPAMIL HCL	PLIVA
AB	No	VERAPAMIL HYDROCHLORIDE	Tablet; Oral	120MG	VERAPAMIL HCL	WATSON LABS
AB	No	VERAPAMIL HYDROCHLORIDE	Tablet; Oral	40MG	VERAPAMIL HCL	WATSON LABS
AB	No	VERAPAMIL HYDROCHLORIDE	Tablet; Oral	80MG	VERAPAMIL HCL	WATSON LABS

Table I - Orange Book (Electronic) Listings (abridged) for Verapamil Hydrochloride Oral Tablets

TE Code	RLD	Active Ingredient	Dosage Form; Route	Strength	Proprietary Name	Applicant
BC	Yes	VERAPAMIL HYDROCHLORIDE	Tablet, Extended Release;Oral	180MG	COVERA-HS	GD SEARLE LLC
BC	Yes	VERAPAMIL HYDROCHLORIDE	Tablet, Extended Release;Oral	240MG	COVERA-HS	GD SEARLE LLC

Table II – Orange Book (Electronic) Listing
(abridged) for Covera-HS Tablets

Table III depicts abridged Electronic Orange Book information concerning 120 mg extended-release oral capsule dosage forms of diltiazem hydrochloride. Note that the Cardizem CD product is the reference standard used by the FDA to compare these products. Note also that some of the products on the chart are labeled AB2 or AB3. AB2 products are bioequivalent to other AB2 diltiazem hydrochloride sustained-release 120mg capsule products but are not bioequivalent with AB3 products. Likewise, AB3 products are bioequivalent with each other but not with AB2 products. If a product was associated with a BC code, it would not be possible to substitute any other products on this chart for this one.

What if a prescriber writes for Mylan's 120 mg extended release capsule? May a pharmacist substitute with Andrx's 120 mg product? Yes, because they are both AB2 rated AND provided that it is less expensive than Mylan's product. This again relates to the fact that ALL drug products containing the exact same drug and dosage form share the same generic name. Generic substitution means that any drug product, whether it has a generic name only or has been given a trade name or brand name, may be used as a substitute, IF it is less expensive.

TE Code	RLD	Active Ingredient	Dosage Form; Route	Strength	Proprietary Name	Applicant
AB2	No	DILTIAZEM HYDROCHLORIDE	Capsule, Extended Release; Oral	120MG	DILTIAZEM HCL	ANDRX
AB3	No	DILTIAZEM HYDROCHLORIDE	Capsule, Extended Release; Oral	120MG	CARTIA XT	ANDRX PHARMS
AB3	Yes	DILTIAZEM HYDROCHLORIDE	Capsule, Extended Release; Oral	120MG	CARDIZEM CD	BIOVAIL
AB3	No	DILTIAZEM HYDROCHLORIDE	Capsule, Extended Release; Oral	120MG	DILTIAZEM HCL	BIOVAIL
AB2	No	DILTIAZEM HYDROCHLORIDE	Capsule, Extended Release; Oral	120MG	DILTIAZEM HCL	MYLAN
AB3	No	DILTIAZEM HYDROCHLORIDE	Capsule, Extended Release; Oral	120MG	DILTIAZEM HCL	PUREPAC PHARM

Table III – Electronic Orange Book listing (abridged)
of diltiazem hydrochloride extended
release oral capsule products.

The principles explained above apply to other dosage forms as well. For example, Table IV depicts Electronic Orange Book listings for phenytoin oral suspension, oral chewable tablets, and phenytoin sodium injectable solution. Note that all of the phenytoin suspension products have the same strength and have the same AB rating, with Dilantin-125 as the reference standard. Therefore all of these products are considered to be bioequivalent to one another. There is only one oral chewable tablet product and one injectable solution product listed. Therefore, no bioequivalent products are available for these.

TE Code	RLD	Active Ingredient	Dosage Form; Route	Strength	Proprietary Name	Applicant
AB	No	PHENYTOIN	Suspension; Oral	125MG/5ML	PHENYTOIN	ALPHARMA
AB	No	PHENYTOIN	Suspension; Oral	125MG/5ML	PHENTYTOIN	MORTON GROVE
AB	Yes	PHENYTOIN	Suspension; Oral	125MG/5ML	DILANTIN-125	PARKE DAVIS
AB	No	PHENYTOIN	Suspension; Oral	125MG/5ML	PHENYTOIN	TARO
AB	No	PHENYTOIN	Suspension; Oral	125MG/5ML	PHENYTOIN	VISTAPHARM
	Yes	PHENYTOIN	Tablet, Chewable; Oral	50MG	DILANTIN	PFIZER PHARMS
AP	No	PHENYTOIN SODIUM	Injectable; Injection	50MG/ML	PHENYTOIN	ELKINS SINN

Table IV – Electronic Orange Book listing (abridged) of phenytoin suspension, tablet, and injectable dosage forms

Most states originally prohibited or discouraged the substitution of sustained-release, delayed-release, and other dosage forms where there may have been bioequivalence problems. However, in some cases, pharmaceutical companies have submitted data showing bioequivalence. The pharmacist must carefully review the data presented in the Orange Book to ascertain the exact status of a drug product.

Sample Questions

1. Which of the following designations indicate that drug products of the same strength and dosage form may be interchangeable?
   I.   A
   II. AB
   III. B
   (A) I only   (B) III only   (C) I & II only
   (D) II & III only   (E) I, II, & III

2.   The Electronic Orange Book uses the abbreviation RLD to indicate
     (A)   a bioequivalence problem
     (B)   no bioequivalence problem
     (C)   the drug product is used as the reference standard
     (D)   the least expensive drug product
     (E)   the drug product that is preferred by most pharmacists for substitution

Answers: (1) C   (2) C

Mailing of Prescription Drugs

There are virtually no restrictions on mailing prescription products via the United States Postal Service (USPS). At one time controlled substances that were narcotics could not be mailed, but that regulation has been eliminated. The USPS still has regulations that prohibit mailing of poisons or alcohol-containing products that could be considered beverages.

USPS regulations do not apply to commercial shippers such as UPS and FedEx. These private companies may establish their own rules for mailing drug products.

Pharmacists who mail prescriptions, especially controlled substances, should package the prescriptions carefully. Any identification on the outside of the package indicating the presence of a prescription drug should be avoided.

Sample Questions

1. The major objective of the Orange Book is to compare drug products that are:
   (A) official in the USP/NF
   (B) multi-source
   (C) chemically unique
   (D) most economical
   (E) therapeutically unique

2. Colonial Labs is the first company to develop and market a particular product as a transdermal patch. This product would probably be described in the Orange Book as:
   I. NTI
   II. A rated
   III. the reference drug product
   (A) I only   (B) III only   (C) I & II only
   (D) II & III only (E) I, II, & III

3. Certain drug products are exempt from the requirements of demonstrating therapeutic equivalence because of:
   I. the grandfather clause
   II. their narrow therapeutic index
   III. their high therapeutic index
   (A) I only   (B) III only   (C) I & II only
   (D) II & III only (E) I, II, & III

4. Major objectives for developing a formulary include
   I. reduce drug inventory
   II. allow therapeutic substitution
   III. give prescribers greater latitude for drug selection
   (A) I only   (B) III only   (C) I & II only
   (D) II & III only (E) I, II, & III

5. Therapeutic substitution is permitted only if an institution is:
   (A) nonprofit
   (B) for profit
   (C) using a formulary system
   (D) under the supervision of a PharmD
   (E) approved to do so by the FDA

6. Substitution is permitted for drug products with which of the following codes?
   I.   A
   II. AB
   III. B
   (A) I only   (B) III only   (C) I & II only
   (D) II & III only   (E) I, II, & III

7. Which of the following reference sources contain(s) significant information concerning bioequivalence of drug products?
   I.   Orange Book
   II. USP DI
   III. USP/NF
   (A) I only   (B) III only   (C) I & II only
   (D) II & III only   (E) I, II, & III

8. Which of the following volumes of the USP DI contains significant information concerning bioequivalence of drug products?
   I.   Volume I
   II.   Volume II
   III. Volume III
   (A) I only   (B) III only   (C) I & II only
   (D) II & III only   (E) I, II, & III

Answers: (1) B (2) B (3) A (4) C (5) C (6) C (7) C
           (8) B

OBRA 90 and Patient Counseling

Portions of OBRA 90 directly impact upon pharmaceutical dispensing and care. The Medicaid Prudent Pharmaceutical Purchasing Provisions of this Act, establishes conditions for the federal government to reimburse states for outpatient Medicaid services. In order for a state to receive money for its Medicaid program, it must have a drug use or drug utilization review (DUR) program. The DUR program must include a prospective component (i.e. one that examines future drug use) and a retrospective program (i.e. one that examines past drug use).

Note

Remember that the Federal Health Care Financing Administration (HCFA) controls and administers Medicare while the individual states administer Medicaid programs.

The prospective DUR is a review of a patient's written medical record and/or his medication profile before dispensing a prescription to the patient. The pharmacist must make a reasonable effort to obtain and update a patient medication profile for every person receiving prescriptions. Minimally, the following information is required in the profile:

- Patient's name, address, telephone number

- Age or date of birth

- The sex of the patient

- Disease state(s) information if known or provided by the patient or their physician

- Any known allergies

- A list of medications previously dispensed

- Pharmacist comments concerning the patient's drug therapy, when appropriate

Patients may refuse to divulge any or all of the above information, but the pharmacist should create or refer to the patient's medication profile and indicate the refusal of the patient to provide information.

When a prescription is presented to the pharmacist, he or she must perform a prospective DUR. This consists of:

- A review of the prescription and patient records for over or under utilization of drugs.

- Checking for therapeutic duplication.

- Checking for incorrect doses or dosing regimens.

- Extending a verbal offer to the client or their representative to personally discuss matters that will enhance or optimize their drug therapy.

A critical portion of OBRA 90 that affects dispensing pharmacists is the requirement that an offer to counsel the patient must be provided. The OBRA 90 legislation specifically provides for patient counseling for Medicaid patients. Since Medicaid is under the jurisdiction of the individual states, each state has the right to establish whether patient counseling will be required for all patients. Most states have taken the realistic stand that all patients should be provided with the opportunity to be counseled. Most state boards of pharmacy have or are in the process of establishing standards of care, which require active verbal offers of counseling, not just a check-off system performed by a clerk.

What type of information must the pharmacist provide if counseling is requested? Federal law does not state how much or what specific information is to be provided by the pharmacist. Instead, pharmacists must use their professional judgment to determine the type and extent of information to provide. Appropriate information could include:

- The name and use of the drug

- The route of administration and duration of the drug therapy

- Any special directions or cautions for taking the drug

- Common adverse effects that may be experienced

- How the patient may evaluate the effectiveness of his/her drug therapy

- How the drug should be stored and when it should be discarded

- Whether the prescription may be refilled

- What the patient should do if a dose is missed

> **Note**
>
> Remember. These are only examples of some of the information that the pharmacist may supply. None of these items is absolutely required and the counseling session could include anything the pharmacist considers necessary. Obviously the pharmacist should always inquire if the patient has further questions.

When does the pharmacist NOT have to counsel a patient? Only if the patient refuses to be counseled.

May a pharmacy intern counsel a patient? The utilization of pharmacy interns to counsel patients is a decision made by each state board of pharmacy. Most have included patient counseling as a function of registered pharmacy interns.

The retrospective drug utilization review is a requirement for individual states. It is not for pharmacies. It is expected that each state will establish a committee consisting of physicians, pharmacists, and other health professsionals. This board or committee reviews the use of certain drugs over a period of time to ascertain whether appropriate therapy is being utilized. Obviously, the retrospective DUR is performed after prescriptions have been dispensed and information concerning the prescriptions has been sent to a clearinghouse - usually the state's Medicaid center. The DUR board may recommend that some prescribing habits of physicians be changed. The board may also initiate educational programs for both physicians and pharmacists.

OBRA 90 also established and funded demonstration projects with the intent of evaluating outcomes of patient care and the cost efficiency of pharmacist interventions.

Another objective of the OBRA 90 legislation was to reduce the cost of state Medicaid programs. Pharmaceutical manufacturers are required to offer Medicaid programs the lowest price ("best price") for drug products. If the price being charged is higher than the price charged to any other group, the company must offer a rebate of the difference to the state Medicaid program.

Health Insurance Portability & Accountability Act (HIPAA)

The basic intent of this act is to assure the security and privacy of patients' medical records while allowing the flow of health information needed to provide high quality health care. Every health care provider who electronically transmits health information is a covered entity. The rule is intended to limit the use, requests for, or disclosure of protected health information (PHI). Pharmacists should be aware that such privacy includes prescriptions, patient record systems (including a patient's prescription profiles) and recorded pharmacist comments relevant to patient therapy. While most states already have regulations concerning the confidentiality of patient medical records, the Federal Act contains substantial fines for breaks in confidentiality.

Medical facilities such as clinics, hospitals, physician offices, etc. must provide a written privacy notice to each patient. This notice describes how medical information concerning the patient may be used and disclosed. It also will advise the patient how he/she can get access to the information. Most facilities will require the patient to sign an acknowledgment that the notice was provided. This signed form must be kept for a minimum of six years, but there is no requirement for future signatures. All medical personnel must be trained by the organization's "HIPAA Privacy Officer" concerning the HIPAA requirements.

The HIPAA "privacy rule" requires that a patient consent to the sharing of private data. Blanket "consent" forms are often used by institutions, etc. to safeguard their rights to information. Also, most insurance companies require that their clients sign a waiver allowing the company to process and audit medical and prescription claims. When information concerning several patients is being accumulated, a "de-indentification" process must be considered. For example, when publishing a research paper or delivering a seminar presentation, the investigator or speaker must remove individual patient names, addresses or other identifying information.

Patients may report perceived violations of the HIPAA requirements to the Department of Health and Human Services Office for Civil Rights (HHS/OCR)

Since pharmacies must also adhere to the HIPAA requirements, patients should be notified about their privacy rights and how their health care information (medical histories and prescriptions records) may be used. The pharmacy must post its entire "Notice of Privacy Practices" in a prominent location within the pharmacy as well as on its web site, if one exists.

When professional service is first initiated with a new patient, the patient must be informed of the privacy provisions used by the pharmacy. Ideally, a written acknowledgment from the patient of receipt of the notice should be obtained, but having the patient sign or initial the prescription log book is acceptable provided the patient is informed of the purpose of the signature.

All family members do not have to receive the notice; instead, just the person named in an insurance policy. Thus, children under the age of 18 are not required to sign the privacy notice. A record of required signatures must be maintained for six years from date obtained or from the last date a prescription is dispensed (whichever is later).

Patient records must be maintained securely. Theoretically, the only parties that should have access to a specific prescription or patient prescription records are the individual patient, the pharmacist and auxiliary personnel authorized to fill or read a prescription, the prescriber and his/her personnel, and authorized legal personnel such as board of pharmacy inspectors or DEA inspectors. While it is obvious that a pharmacist should not allow pharm-aceutical sales representatives or other individuals to ran-domly review the pharmacy's prescription files or a medication profile, other situations are more complex. For example, can the spouse of a patient see the medication profile or receive a copy of the prescription? Theoretically, the actual patient must grant written permission first.

If a pharmacy mails a friendly reminder to a patient concerning the need for a refill of a prescription, it should be done in a manner in which others will not see the drug name or therapeutic use. The name of a drug or its use should not be given upon telephone request unless the pharmacist is certain that the patient has agreed to the request.

Consultations with the patient concerning prescriptions must be conducted in a manner that minimizes the likelihood of incidental disclosures to other persons who may be nearby. Communications over the telephone should be conducted so that unauthorized persons will not overhear conversations. It is permissible to leave messages on answering machines or with a family member provided only "minimally necessary" information is provided. It is also permissible for the pharmacist using his/her professsional judgment to allow a relative or friend to pick up a filled prescription. It is not necessary for the patient to provide written permission or give the name of the person picking up the prescription in advance.

International Commerce Involving Drugs and Drug Products

Laws and regulations for the transportation of drugs and drug products between the United States and foreign countries are both confusing and subject to change by the Congress, FDA, or the Executive administration. Three terms often employed, but with somewhat ambiguous definitions, are exportation, importation, and reimportation of drug products. This book will use the following definitions:

Exportation is the shipment of drug products to a foreign country. This action will be acceptable if performed by the original manufacturer or a duly licensed wholesaler, and there is no intention to bring the product back into the United States.

Importation implies that a drug product is being brought into the United States for distribution. Theoretically the drug product must meet all of the standards established by the FDA for that drug including the FDA's GMP and labeling standards.

Reimportation refers to a drug product that is manufactured in the United States with FDA-approved labeling, shipped to a foreign country, and then shipped back into the United States. According to the FDA, this procedure is legal only if performed by the original manufacturer.

Out-of-state and Foreign Prescriptions

Controversial issues relate to the legality of pharmacists filling prescriptions written by prescribers in other states and in foreign countries and Americans who obtain prescription drugs from other countries.

The legality of filling of prescriptions written by prescribers in other states or foreign countries is not a clear legal issue. Most individual states have regulations, which define which health professionals may diagnose, treat, dispense, and prescribe. Often the regulations specify that only liensed practitioners may write prescriptions with the understanding that pharmacies will fill only those prescriptions written within the state. However, current practice often entails filling out-of-state prescriptions. The prime consideration for the pharmacist is to establish that the prescriber, the patient and the prescription are legitimate. Using his/her professional judgment, the pharmacist should ascertain the legitimacy of each prescription received.

The federal government has not taken a clear stand on prescriptions written in foreign countries by prescribers who are not licensed in the United States. The power to control such prescriptions has been left mainly to the individual states. Some states, especially those bordering foreign countries or with a large number of foreign visitors, allow the filling of foreign prescriptions. As usual, the pharmacist must use his/her professional judgment in deciding which prescriptions to fill.

A side issue relates to whether a pharmacy may fill a foreign prescription and directly export it to a foreign country. This appears to be legitimate if the prescription is for a reasonable quantity of drug. Conversely, a person in this country can import reasonable supplies of a prescription drug. It should be remembered that prescription drugs must be used under the supervision of a prescriber. In filling foreign prescriptions or mailing drug products to other countries it becomes difficult for the pharmacist to determine whether or not a patient is being properly monitored.

Note

NONE of the above statements apply to controlled substances. Federal regulations require that only practitioners licensed to practice in the United States may write prescriptions for controlled substances.

Another current issue is the practice of some individuals who obtain prescription drugs from outside the United States via the mail or by visiting another country. The FDA does not sanction such actions but appears to allow importation of drug products for personal use provided:

1. The patient declares that the drug product is for his/her personal use and identifies the practitioner under whose care it will be used.

2. The quantity is not excessive, which is usually defined as not more than a three month supply.

3. The use for the drug product is clearly identified.

4. The drug product will not be distributed to others.

The drug supply may be shipped directly to the patient or to either his/her physician or pharmacy.

In addition, the FDA has stated that businesses such as internet pharmacies must sell only FDA-approved drugs, including those manufactured in foreign countries. This means that the drug product must meet ALL FDA standards for manufacturing, ingredients, formulations, etc.

The FDA has also established a policy of allowing small quantities of drug products that are sold abroad to be brought into the United States, provided they are used for patient treatment of serious conditions for which effective treatment may not be otherwise available.

Sample Questions

1. What constitutes appropriate action for a pharmacist when an uncooperative patient refuses to provide information for his patient prescription profile?
   I.   The pharmacist may refuse to fill the prescription.
   II. The pharmacist may fill the prescription without a medication history.
   III. The pharmacist should explain that it is illegal for the patient to refuse to provide the requested information.
   (A) I only   (B) III only   (C) I & II only
   (D) II & III only   (E) I, II, & III

2. Which of the following might represent a breach of privacy based upon the federal Health Insurance Portability and Accountability Act (HIPAA)
    I.   Allowing a pharmaceutical sales representative to peruse your prescription files to ascertain if a certain doctor is prescribing his company's new antidepressant.
    II.   Sending a postcard reminding a patient that his Prozac prescription needs to be refilled.
    III. Providing a husband with a list of drug products and their therapeutic uses, that his wife received last year.
    (A) I only   (B) III only   (C) I & II only
    (D) II & III only   (E) I, II, & III

3. According to FDA guidelines, which of the following activities are NOT acceptable for an individual receiving mailed prescription drug products from a Canadian pharmacy?
    I.   Splitting the drug supply with his neighbor who has a prescription for the same product
    II.   Receiving a six months supply of the drug product
    III. Having the drug mailed directly to his home rather than to his physician
    (A) I only   (B) III only   (C) I & II only
    (D) II & III only   (E) I, II, & III

4. A police officer visits a pharmacy and informs the pharmacist that he has arrested an individual suspected of writing a fictitious prescription that was filled in the pharmacy. The officer requests the original prescription as evidence. Which of the following would be appropriate actions for the pharmacist to take?

I. The pharmacist should give the officer the prescription as long as he provides a written receipt.
II. As described, the prescription is not legally considered to be a forged prescription.
III. The pharmacist is not obligated to give the officer the prescription.

(A) I only   (B) III only   (C) I & II only
(D) II & III only   (E) I, II, & III

5. Under the Poison Prevention Packaging Act (PPPA), the use of closures that are "reversible", i.e. not child-resistant in one direction but child-resistant in the opposite position is
   (A) permitted only for use in prescriptions intended for geriatric patients
   (B) discouraged but not prohibited under the PPA
   (C) illegal
   (D) permitted only for use in nursing homes
   (E) permitted only for use in hospice patients

6. A client presents a prescription for an antidiabetic drug written for his cousin living in France. Which one of the following actions is MOST appropriate for the pharmacist to take?
   (A) Refuse to fill the prescription stating that the condition is not life-threatening
   (B) Fill the prescription after obtaining a written guarantee that the drug will be shipped abroad
   (C) Fill the prescription using professional judgment to determine that it is a legitimate prescription
   (D) Refuse to fill the prescription stating that both federal and state laws prohibits such dispensing
   (E) Fill the prescription after obtaining permission from the FDA

Answers: (1) C   (2) E   (3) C   (4) D   (5) B   (6) C

Section G

Controlled Substances

Definitions Related to Controlled Substances

The following definitions are listed in the Controlled Substances Act (CSA). While candidates are not required to write out definitions on the MPJE®, they are expected to be able to understand these terms when they are used in questions. Of particular importance are definitions that include lists of drugs. Candidates should review these lists carefully and be able to identify drugs listed in questions. Candidates should not try to memorize any of these definitions, but review them so they are somewhat familiar.

ACT - the Controlled Substances Act and/or the Controlled Substances Import and Export Act as amended periodically.

ADDICT -any individual who habitually uses any narcotic drug so as to endanger the public morals, health, safety, or welfare, or who is so far addicted to the use of narcotic drugs as to have lost the power of self-control with reference to his addiction.

Note

A person who becomes habituated while using a prescribed narcotic is not generally considered to be an addict.

ADMINISTRATION - the Drug Enforcement Administration.

ADMINISTRATOR - the Administrator of the Drug Enforcement Administration (DEA). The Administrator has been delegated authority under the Act by the Attorney General.

ANABOLIC STEROID - any drug or hormonal substance, chemically and pharmacologically related to testosterone (other than estrogens, progestins, and corticosteroids) that promotes muscle growth, and includes:

- Boldenone
- Chlorotestosterone (4-chlortestosterone)
- Clostebol
- Dehydrochlormethyltestosterone
- Dihydrotestosterone (4-dihydrotestosterone)
- Drostanolone
- Ethylestrenol
- Fluoxymesterone
- Formebulone (formebolone)
- Mesterolone
- Methandienone
- Methandranone
- Methandriol
- Methandrostenolone
- Methenolone
- Methyltestosterone

- Mibolerone
- Nandrolone
- Norethandrolone
- Oxandrolone
- Oxymesterone
- Oxymetholone
- Stanolone
- Stanozolol
- Testolactone
- Testosterone
- Trenbolone
- Any salt, ester, or isomer of a drug or substance described or listed above, if that salt, ester, or isomer promotes muscle growth. Except such terms do not include an anabolic steroid which is expressly intended for administration through implants to cattle or other non-human species and which has been approved by the Secretary of Health and Human Services for such administration. If any per-son prescribes, dispenses, or distributes such steroid for human use, such person shall be considered to have prescribed, dispensed, or distributed an anabolic steroid within the meaning of this paragraph.

Study Tip

Most drugs that have anabolic steroid activity have the suffix "androlone" in them. Look for that suffix in questions related to these drugs.

COMMERCIAL CONTAINER - any bottle, jar, tube, ampule, or other receptacle in which a substance is held for distribution or dispensing to an ultimate user, or held for distribution or dispensing to an ultimate user. The term commercial container does not include any package liner, package insert or other material kept with or within a commercial container, nor any carton, crate, drum, or other package in which commercial containers are stored or are used for shipment of controlled substances.

COMPOUNDER - any person engaging in maintenance or detoxification treatment who also mixes, prepares, packages or changes the dosage form of a narcotic drug listed in Schedules II, III, IV or V for use in maintenance or detoxification treatment by another narcotic treatment program.

DETOXIFICATION TREATMENT - the dispensing, for a period of time as specified below, of a narcotic drug or narcotic drugs in decreasing doses to an individual to alleviate adverse physiological or psychological effects as part of their withdrawal from the continuous or sustained use of a narcotic drug. Such programs are intended to bring the individual to a narcotic drug-free state within such period of time. There are two types of detoxification treatment, short-term detoxification treatment and long-term detoxification treatment.

- Short-term detoxification treatment is for a period not in excess of 30 days.

- Long-term detoxification treatment is for a period more than 30 days but not in excess of 180 days.

DISPENSER - an individual practitioner, institutional practitioner, pharmacy or pharmacist who dispenses a controlled substance.

DRUG - (A) articles recognized in the official United States Pharmacopoeia, official Homoeopathic Pharmacopoeia of the United States, or official National Formulary, or any supplement to any of them; and (B) articles intended for use in the diagnosis, cure, mitigation, treatment, or prevention of disease in man or other animals; and (C) articles (other than food) intended to affect the structure or any function of the body of man or other animals;

EXPORT - taking out or removal of drugs listed in the CSA from the jurisdiction of the United States.

EXPORTER - includes every person who exports, or who acts as an export broker for exportation of controlled substances listed in any schedule.

HEARING - (A) Any hearing held for the granting, denial, revocation, or suspension of a registration; or (B) Any hearing held to set quotas for the amount of controlled substance that may be purchased or manufactured; or (C) Any hearing held for the issuance, amendment, or repeal of any rule issued as part of the Controlled Substances Act.

IMPORT - bringing in or introduction of a controlled substance into either the jurisdiction of the United States or the customs territory of the United States.

IMPORTER - includes every person who imports, or who acts as an import broker for importation of controlled substances listed in any schedule.

INDIVIDUAL PRACTITIONER - a physician, dentist, veterinarian, or other individual licensed, registered, or otherwise permitted, by the United States or the jurisdiction in which he/she practices, to dispense a controlled substance in the course of professional practice. This term does not include a pharmacist, a pharmacy, or an institutional practitioner.

INSTITUTIONAL PRACTITIONER - a hospital or other entity (other than an individual) licensed, registered, or otherwise permitted, by the United States or the jurisdiction in which it practices, to dispense a controlled substance in the course of professional practice. This term does not include a pharmacy.

INVENTORY - all stocks of Schedule I or II controlled substances manufactured or otherwise acquired by a registrant, whether in bulk, commercial containers, or contained in pharmaceutical preparations and that are in the possession of the registrant.

JURISDICTION OF THE UNITED STATES - the customs territory of the United States, the Virgin Islands, the Canal Zone, Guam, American Samoa, and the Trust Territories of the Pacific Islands.

LABEL - any display of written, printed, or graphic matter placed upon the commercial container of any controlled substance by its manufacturer.

LABELING - all labels and other written, printed, or graphic matter on any controlled substance or any of its commercial containers or wrappers. This also includes such material that accompanies such a controlled substance.

LISTED CHEMICAL - any List I chemical or List II chemical. (see below for further clarification)

LIST I CHEMICAL - A chemical specifically identified in the CSA that, in addition to legitimate uses, is used in manufacturing a controlled substance in violation of the Act and is important to the manufacture of a controlled substance (e.g. ergotamine, phenylpropanolamine).

LIST II CHEMICAL - a chemical, other than a List I chemical that, in addition to legitimate uses, is used in manufacturing a controlled substance in violation of the Act (e.g. acetone, ethyl ether)

LONG TERM CARE FACILITY (LTCF) - a nursing home, retirement care, mental care or other facility or institution which provides extended health care to resident patients.

MAINTENANCE TREATMENT - the dispensing, for a period in excess of twenty-one days, of a narcotic drug or narcotic drugs in the treatment of an individual for dependence upon heroin or other morphine-like drug.

MANUFACTURE

- The producing, preparation, propagation, compounding, manufacturing, or processing of a drug or other substance.

- The packaging or repackaging of such substance.

- The labeling or re-labeling of the commercial container of such substance.

This definition does not include the activities of a practitioner who administers, dispenses, prepares, compounds, packages or labels such substance in the course of his/her professional practice.

MID-LEVEL PRACTITIONER - an individual practitioner, OTHER than a physician, dentist, veterinarian, or podiatrist, who is licensed, registered, or otherwise permitted by the United States or the jurisdiction in which he/she practices, to dispense a controlled substance in the course of professional practice.

Note

Examples of mid-level practitioners include, but are not limited to, health care providers such as nurse practitioners, nurse midwives, nurse anesthetists, clinical nurse specialists and physician assistants who are authorized to dispense controlled substances by the state in which they practice.

NAME - the official, brand, common, chemical or usual name of a substance.

NARCOTIC DRUG - any of the following drugs, no matter how they are derived or synthesized:

- Opium, opiates, derivatives of opium and opiates, including their isomers, esters, ethers, salts, and salts of isomers, esters, and ethers. Such term does not include the isoquinoline alkaloids of opium.

- Poppy straw and concentrate of poppy straw.

- Coca leaves, *except* coca leaves and extracts of coca leaves from which cocaine, ecgonine and derivatives of ecgonine or their salts have been removed.

- Cocaine, its salts, optical and geometric isomers, and salts of isomers.

- Ecgonine, its derivatives, their salts, isomers and salts of isomers.

- Any compound, mixture, or preparation which contains any quantity of any of the substances referred to in this section.

NARCOTIC TREATMENT PROGRAM - a program engaged in maintenance and/or detoxification treatment with narcotic drugs.

NET DISPOSAL - for a stated period, the quantity of a Schedule I or II controlled substance distributed by the registrant to another person, plus the quantity of that substance used by the registrant in the production of (or converted by the registrant into) another Schedule I or II controlled or noncontrolled substance, plus the quantity of such drugs that are disposed of by the registrant. This quantity is reduced by any Schedule I or II drugs returned to the registrant by any purchaser, and distributed by the registrant to another registered manufacturer.

PHARMACIST - any pharmacist licensed by a state to dispense controlled substances, and any other person (e.g., a pharmacy intern) authorized by a state to dispense controlled substances under the supervision of a pharmacist licensed by such State.

PERSON - any individual, corporation, government or governmental subdivision or agency, business trust, partnership, association, or other legal entity.

PRESCRIPTION - an order for medication which is dispensed to an ultimate user. This definition does not include an order for medication dispensed for immediate administration to a patient. (e.g., an order to dispense a drug for immediate administration to an inpatient in a hospital is not a prescription.)

PURCHASER - any registered person entitled to obtain and execute order forms pursuant to the CSA.

READILY RETRIEVABLE - records that are kept in such a manner that they can be separated out from all other records in a reasonable time.

REGISTER (REGISTRATION) - refers only to registration required and permitted by the Controlled Substances Act.

REGISTRANT - any person who is registered under the Controlled Substance Act.

SUPPLIER - any registered person entitled to fill order forms under the Controlled Substances Act.

Registration of Manufacturers, Distributors, and Dispensers

Individuals (e.g. researchers), manufacturers, distributors, laboratories, exporters, narcotic treatment programs, or dispensing locations (e.g. pharmacies), who are authorized to possess controlled substances, must be registered by the DEA to engage in these activities.

> # Note
> Pharmacists do not generally need to register with the DEA if they are working in a registered establishment.

At the time a retail pharmacy, hospital/clinic, practitioner or teaching institution is first registered, that business activity shall be assigned to a specific month of the year. The expiration date of the registrant will be the last day of the month designated. After the initial registration period, the registration expires 36 months from the initial expiration date.

Applications for Registration

Specific DEA registration forms must be used by different types of entities to register with the DEA, for example:
- Pharmacies – Form 224
- Manufacturers or Researchers – Form 225
- Narcotic Treatment Programs - Form 363

Registration renewal forms for these entities generally have the same number, but with an "a" suffix, i.e. 224a, 225a, and 363a. These forms are mailed to each registered entity approximately 60 days before the expiration date of the registration.

If a registered entity does not receive registration renewal forms within 45 days before the expiration date of his/her registration, he/she must promptly notify DEA and request such forms in writing.

Note

Remember these important time periods:

- A DEA registration is valid for 36 months
- Registration renewal forms are sent to the registrant 60 days before the expiration date of the registration.
- Registrants must notify DEA in writing if they have not received their renewal forms within 45 days of their expiration date.

Each application must include all information called for in the form, unless the item is not applicable, in which case this fact shall be indicated.

Each application, attachment, or other document filed as part of an application, must be signed by the

- applicant, if an individual
- by a partner of the applicant, if a partnership
- or by an officer of the applicant, if a corporation, corporate division, association, trust or other entity

An applicant may authorize one or more individuals, who would not otherwise be authorized to do so, to sign applications for the applicant by filing with the Registration Unit of the DEA a Power of Attorney for each such individual. A person who is authorized to sign registration applications must sign the Power of Attorney. It must also contain the signature of the individual being authorized to sign applications. The Power of Attorney is valid until revoked by the applicant.

Note

Every location where controlled substances are manufactured, distributed or dispensed must have its own DEA registration EXCEPT for the following:

- Warehouses used by registrants to store controlled substances.
- A practitioner's office where drugs are prescribed, but not administered or dispensed.
- Common carriers (e.g. freight delivery companies)
- An office where sales of controlled substances are solicited, made or supervised, but the location does not contain controlled substances.

Re-registration

Any person who is registered may apply to be re-registered not more than 60 days before the expiration date of his/her registration. Bulk manufacturers of Schedule I or II controlled substances or importers of Schedule I or II controlled substances may apply to be re-registered not more than 120 days before the expiration date of their registration.

Commercial Containers

Each commercial container containing a controlled substance must have printed on the label the symbol designating the product's assigned controlled substance schedule (i.e. C-II, C-III, etc). The word "Schedule" need not be used. The symbol must be large enough to be easily seen without taking the container off the shelf.

Schedule I Controlled Substances

Drugs classified as Schedule I controlled substances are those that have the following characteristics:

- have a high potential for abuse
- have no currently accepted medical use in treatment in the United States
- lack accepted information on the safety of their use, even under medical supervision

Included in Schedule I are the following drugs or substances:

- Opiates. Unless specifically excepted or unless listed in another schedule, any of the following opiates, including their isomers, esters, ethers, salts, and salts of isomers, esters and ethers:

    (1) Acetyl-alpha-methylfentanyl(N-[1-(1-methyl-2-phenethyl)-4-piperidinyl]-N-phenylacetamide
    (2) Acetylmethadol
    (3) Allylprodine
    (4) Alphacetylmethadol(except levoalphacetyl-methadol also known as levo-alpha-acetylmethadol, levomethadyl acetate, or LAAM)
    (5) Alphameprodine
    (6) Alphamethadol
    (7) Alpha-methylfentanyl(N-[1-(alpha-methyl-beta-phenyl)ethyl-4-piperidyl]propionanilide;1-(1-methyl-2-phenyl-ethyl)-4-(N-propanilido) piperidine

(8) Alpha-methylthiofentanyl(N-[1-methyl-2-(2-thienyl)ethyl-4-piperidinyl]-N-phenyl-propanamide

(9) Benzethidine

(10) Betacetylmethadol

(11) Beta-hydroxyfentanyl(N-[1-(2-hydroxy-2-phenethyl)-4-piperidinyl]-N-phenyl-propanamide

(12) Beta-hydroxy-3-methylfentanyl(other name: N-[1-(2-hydroxy-2-phenethyl)-3-methyl-4-piperidinyl]-N-phenyl-propanamide

(13) Betameprodine

(14) Betamethadol

(15) Betaprodine

(16) Clonitazene

(17) Dextromoramide

(18) Diampromide

(19) Diethylthiambutene

(20) Difenoxin

(21) Dimenoxadol

(22) Dimepheptanol

(23) Dimethylthiambutene

(24) Dioxaphetyl butyrate

(25) Dipipanone

(26) Ethylmethylthiambutene

(27) Etonitazene

(28) Etoxeridine

(29) Furethidine

(30) Hydroxypethidine

(31) Ketobemidone

(32) Levomoramide

(33) Levophenacylmorphan

(34) 3-Methylfentanyl(N-[3-methyl-1-(2-phenylethyl)-4-piperidyl]-N-phenyl-propanamide

(35) 3-methylthiofentanyl(N-[(3-methyl-1-(2-thienyl)ethyl-4-piperidinyl]-N-phenyl-propanamide)

(36)   Morpheridine
(37)   MPPP(1-methyl-4-phenyl-4-propion-oxy-
             piperidine
(38)   Noracymethadol
(39)   Norlevorphanol
(40)   Normethadone
(41)   Norpipanone
(42)   Para-fluorofentanyl(N-(4-fluorophenyl)-N-[1-
             (2-phenethyl)-4-piperidinyl] propan-amide
(43)   PEPAP(1-(-2-phenethyl)-4-phenyl-4-acetoxy-
             piperidine
(44)   Phenadoxone
(45)   Phenampromide
(46)   Phenomorphan
(47)   Phenoperidine
(48)   Piritramide
(49)   Proheptazine
(50)   Properidine
(51)   Propiram
(52)   Racemoramide
(53)   Thiofentanyl(N-phenyl-N-[1-(2-
             thienyl)ethyl-4-piperidinyl]- propanamide
(54)   Tilidine
(55)   Trimeperidine

- Opium derivatives. Unless specifically excepted or unless listed in another schedule, any of the following opium derivatives, its salts, isomers, and salts of isomers:

(1)   Acetorphine
(2)   Acetyldihydrocodeine
(3)   Benzylmorphine
(4)   Codeine methylbromide
(5)   Codeine-N-Oxide

(6)   Cyprenorphine
(7)   Desomorphine
(8)   Dihydromorphine
(9)   Drotebanol
(10)   Etorphine (except hydrochloride salt)
(11)   Heroin
(12)   Hydromorphinol
(13)   Methyldesorphine
(14)   Methyldihydromorphine
(15)   Morphine methylbromide
(16)   Morphine methylsulfonate
(17)   Morphine-N-Oxide
(18)   Myrophine
(19)   Nicocodeine
(20)   Nicomorphine
(21)   Normorphine
(22)   Pholcodine
(23)   Thebacon

- Hallucinogenic substances. Unless specifically excepted or unless listed in another schedule, any material, compound, mixture, or preparation, which contains any quantity of the following hallucinogenic substances, or which contains any of its salts, isomers, and salts of isomers:

(1)   alpha-ethyltryptamine(etryptamine; Monase, AET)
(2)   4-bromo-2,5-dimethoxy-amphetamine(4-bromo-2,5-DMA)
(3)   4-bromo-2,5-dimethoxyphenethylamine(2C-B, Nexus)
(4)   2,5-dimethoxyamphetamine (2,5-DMA)
(5)   2,5-dimethoxy-4-ethylamphet-amine (DOET)
(6)   4-methoxyamphetamine paramethoxy-amphetamine, PMA)
(7)   5-methoxy-3,4-mdthylenedioxy-amphetamine

   (8)   4-methyl-2,5-dimethoxy-amphetamine("DOM"
         and "STP")
   (9)   3,4-methylenedioxy amphetamine
 (10)   3,4-methylenedioxymethamphetamine (MDMA)
 (11)   3,4-methylenedioxy-N-ethylamphetamine(N-ethyl
         MDA, MDE, MDEA)
 (12)   N-hydroxy-3,4-methylenedioxy-amphetamine (N-
         hydroxy MDA)
 (13)   3,4,5-trimethoxy amphetamine
 (14)   Bufotenine (mappine)
 (15)   Diethyltryptamine (DET)
 (16)   Dimethyltryptamine (DMT)
 (17)   Ibogaine (Tabernanthe iboga)
 (18)   Lysergic acid diethylamide (LSD)
 (19)   Marijuana
 (20)   Mescaline
 (21)   Parahexyl (Synhexyl)
 (22)   Peyote
 (23)   N-ethyl-3-piperidyl benzilate
 (24)   N-methyl-3-piperidyl benzilate
 (25)   Psilocybin
 (26)   Psilocyn
 (27)   Tetrahydrocannabinols (THC)
 (28)   Ethylamine analog of phencyclidine (PCE)
 (29)   Pyrrolidine analog of phencyclidine (PCPy,
         PHP)
 (30)   Thiophene analog of phencyclidine (TPCP, TCP)
 (31)   1-[1-(2-thienyl)cyclohexyl]pyrrolidine: (TCPy)

- Depressants. Unless specifically excepted or unless list-
ed in another schedule, any material, compound, mix-
ture, or preparation which contains any quantity of the
following substances having a depressant effect on the
central nervous system, including its salts, isomers, and
salts of isomers.

(1) Gamma-hydroxybutyric acid (GHB)
(2) Mecloqualone
(3) Methaqualone

- Stimulants. Unless specifically excepted or unless listed in another schedule, any material, compound, mixture, or preparation which contains any quantity of the following substances having a stimulant effect on the central nervous system, including its salts, isomers, and salts of isomers:
(1) Aminorex
(2) Cathinone
(3) Fenethylline
(4) Methcathinone (AL-464; AL-422; AL-463 and
        UR1432)
(5) (+/-)cis-4-methylaminorex((+/-)cis-4,5-dihydro-4-
        methyl-5-phenyl-2-oxazolamine)
(6) N-ethylamphetamine
(7) N,N-dimethylamphetamine

- Temporary listing of substances subject to emergency scheduling. Any material, compound, mixture or preparation which contains any quantity of the following substances:

(1) N-[1-benzyl-4-piperidyl]-N-phenylpropanamide
        (benzylfentanyl), its optical isomers, salts and
        salts of isomers

(2) N-[1-(2-thienyl)methyl-4-piperidyl]-N-phenyl-
        propanamide(thenylfentanyl), its optical
        isomers, salts and salts of isomers

Study Tip

Do not attempt to memorize this list! Review it a few times and identify drugs that you may be familiar with (e.g. marijuana, LSD, heroin, mescaline). These are the drugs that you will most likely be questioned about.

Schedule II Controlled Substances

Drugs classified as Schedule II controlled substances are those that have the following characteristics:

- Have a high potential for abuse.
- Have currently accepted medical use in treatment in the United States or a currently accepted medical use with severe restrictions.
- Abuse of the drug or other substance may lead to severe physical or psychological dependence.

Included in Schedule II are the following drugs or substances:

- Opium and any salt, compound, derivative, or preparation of opium excluding apomorphine, thebaine-derived butorphanol, dextrorphan, nalbuphine, nalmefene, naloxone, and naltrexone, and their respective salts, but including the following:
  (1) Raw opium
  (2) Opium extracts
  (3) Opium fluid

    (4)   Powdered opium
    (5)   Granulated opium
    (6)   Tincture of opium
    (7)   Codeine
    (8)   Dihydroetorphine
    (9)   Ethylmorphine
    (10) Etorphine hydrochloride
    (11) Hydromorphone
    (12) Hydrocodone
    (13) Metopon
    (14) Morphine
    (15) Oxycodone
    (16) Oxymorphone
    (17) Thebaine

- Any salt, compound, derivative, or preparation thereof which is chemically equivalent or identical with any of the substances referred to above, except that these substances shall not include the isoquinoline alkaloids of opium.

- Opium poppy and poppy straw

- Coca leaves and any salt, compound, derivative or preparation of coca leaves (including cocaine and ecgonine derivatives).

- Concentrate of poppy straw (the crude extract of poppy straw in either liquid, solid or powder form which contains the phenanthrene alkaloids of the opium poppy

- Opiates. Unless specifically excepted or unless in another schedule any of the following opiates and their derivatives with the exception of dextrorphan and levo-propoxyphene:
  (1)   Alfentanil
  (2)   Alphaprodine
  (3)   Anileridine

    (4)   Bezitramide
    (5)   Bulk dextropropoxyphene (non-dosage forms)
    (6)   Carfentanil
    (7)   Dihydrocodeine
    (8)   Diphenoxylate
    (9)   Fentanyl
    (10)   Isomethadone
    (11)   Levo-alphacetylmethadol(levo-alpha-acetyl-methadol, levomethadyl acetate, LAAM]
    (12)   Levomethorphan
    (13)   Levorphanol
    (14)   Metazocine
    (15)   Methadone
    (16)   Methadone-Intermediate, 4-cyano-2-dimethyl-amino-4,4-diphenyl butane
    (17)   Moramide-Intermediate, 2-methyl-3-morpholino-1, 1-diphenylpropane-carboxylic acid
    (18)   Pethidine (meperidine)
    (19)   Pethidine-Intermediate-A, 4-cyano-1-methyl-4-phenylpiperidine
    (20)   Pethidine-Intermediate-B, ethyl-4-phenyl-piperidine-4-carboxylate
    (21)   Pethidine-Intermediate-C, 1-methyl-4-phenyl-piperidine-4-carboxylic acid
    (22)   Phenazocine
    (23)   Piminodine
    (24)   Racemethorphan
    (25)   Racemorphan
    (26)   Remifentanil
    (27)   Sufentanil

- Stimulants. Unless specifically excepted or unless listed in another schedule, any material, compound, mixture, or preparation which contains any quantity of the following substances having a stimulant effect on the central nervous system:

(1) Amphetamine, its salts, optical isomers, and salts of its optical isomers
(2) Methamphetamine, its salts, isomers, and salts of its isomers
(3) Phenmetrazine and its salts
(4) Methylphenidate

- Depressants. Unless specifically excepted or unless listed in another schedule, any material, compound, mixture, or preparation which contains any quantity of the following substances having a depressant effect on the central nervous system, including its salts, isomers, and salts of isomers.
  (1) Amobarbital
  (2) Glutethimide
  (3) Pentobarbital
  (4) Phencyclidine
  (5) Secobarbital

- Hallucinogenic substances.
  (1) Nabilone

- Immediate precursors. Unless specifically excepted or unless listed in another schedule, any material, compound, mixture, or preparation which contains any quantity of the following substances:
  (1) Immediate precursor to amphetamine and methamphetamine: Phenylacetone
  (2) Immediate precursors to phencyclidine (PCP):
    - 1-phenylcyclohexylamine
    - 1-piperidinocyclohexanecarbonitrile (PCC)

Study Tip

Carefully review the drugs in Schedule II. While some are quite obscure, many are commonly used and are often a source of questions on licensing exams. Remember that Schedule II includes straight opiates and opioids (e.g. codeine, morphine, meperidine) as well as most amphetamines and many barbiturates.

Schedule III Controlled Substances

Drugs classified as Schedule III controlled substances are those that have the following characteristics:

- Have a potential for abuse less than that of the drugs or other substances in schedules I and II.
- Have a currently accepted medical use in treatment in the United States
- Abuse of the drug or other substance may lead to moderate or low physical dependence or high psychological dependence

Included in Schedule III are the following drugs or substances:

- Stimulants. Unless specifically excepted or unless listed in another schedule, any material, compound, mixture, or preparation which contains any quantity of the following substances having a stimulant effect on the central nervous system, including its salts, isomers, and salts of such isomers:

(1) Benzphetamine
(2) Chlorphentermine
(3) Clortermine
(5) Phendimetrazine

- Depressants. Unless specifically excepted or unless listed in another schedule, any material, compound, mixture, or preparation which contains any quantity of the following substances having a depressant effect on the central nervous system:

  (1) Any compound, mixture or preparation containing amobarbital, secobarbital, pentobarbital or any salt thereof and one or more other active medicinal ingredients that are not listed in any schedule.

  (2) Any suppository dosage form containing amobarbital, secobarbital or pentobarbital or any salt of any of these drugs and approved by the Food and Drug Administration for marketing only as a suppository.

Note

Notice that Schedule II barbiturates such as amobarbital, secobarbital, and pentobarbital become Schedule III substances if they are combined with noncontrolled drugs (e.g. aspirin) or if they are in a suppository dosage form.

  (3) Any substance which contains any quantity of a derivative of barbituric acid or any salt thereof
  (4) Any product that contains gamma-hydroxybutyric acid or its derivatives.
  (5) Chlorhexadol

(6)   Ketamine and its derivatives

(7)   Lysergic acid

(8)   Lysergic acid amide

(9)   Methyprylon

(10)   Sulfondiethylmethane

(11)   Sulfonethylmethane

(12)   Sulfonmethane

(13)   Tiletamine and zolazepam (Telazol) or any salt
       thereof

- Nalorphine

- Gamma hydroxybutyrate (GHB, sodium oxybate, Xyrem) – Because of the great abuse potential for this drug, penalties for its illicit use are similar to those for illicit use of Schedule I drugs. The manufacturer of this product has initiated the Xyrem Success Program, which is actually two programs, one directed at the patient and one for the prescriber. Both programs are designed to decrease the likelihood of misuse and diversion of this drug.

- Narcotic Drugs. Unless specifically excepted or unless listed in another schedule, any material, compound, mixture, or preparation containing any of the following narcotic drugs, or their salts calculated as the free anhydrous base or alkaloid, in limited quantities as set forth below:

(1)   Not more than 1.8 grams of codeine per 100 milliliters or not more than 90 milligrams per dosage unit, with an equal or greater quantity of an isoquinoline alkaloid of opium

(2)   Not more than 1.8 grams of codeine per 100 milliliters or not more than 90 milligrams per dosage unit, with one or more active, non-narcotic ingredients in recognized therapeutic amounts

(3)   Not more than 300 milligrams of dihydrocodeinone (hydrocodone) per 100 milliliters or not more than 15 milligrams per dosage unit, with a fourfold or greater quantity of an isoquinoline alkaloid of opium

(4)   Not more than 300 milligrams of dihydrocodeinone (hydrocodone) per 100 milliliters or not more than 15 milligrams per dosage unit, with one or more active non-narcotic ingredients in recognized therapeutic amounts

(5)   Not more than 1.8 grams of dihydrocodeine per 100 milliliters or not more than 90 milligrams per dosage unit, with one or more active non-narcotic ingredients in recognized therapeutic amounts

(6)   Not more than 300 milligrams of ethylmorphine per 100 milliliters or not more than 15 milligrams per dosage unit, with one or more active, non-narcotic ingredients in recognized therapeutic amounts

(7)   Not more than 500 milligrams of opium per 100 milliliters or per 100 grams or not more than 25 milligrams per dosage unit, with one or more active, non-narcotic ingredients in recognized therapeutic amounts

(8)   Not more than 50 milligrams of morphine per 100 milliliters or per 100 grams, with one or more active, non-narcotic ingredients in recognized therapeutic amounts

> ## Study Tip
> Note that with the exception of opium and morphine, quantities of drugs listed in the above section as Schedule III substances are all evenly divisible by 3. This may be helpful if you are asked to determine the Schedule of a compounded product.

- Anabolic steroids. Unless specifically excepted or unless listed in another schedule, any material, compound, mixture, or preparation containing any quantity of anabolic steroids, including their salts, isomers, and salts of isomers

> ## Note
> Anabolic steroids are classified in Schedule III by the federal government. Some states may classify them or other Schedule III substances in Schedule II.

- Buprenorphine (Subutex)

- Buprenorphine + naloxone (Suboxone)

Schedule IV Controlled Substances

Drugs classified as schedule IV controlled substances are those that have the following characteristics:

- Have a low potential for abuse relative to the drugs or other substances in schedule III.

- Have a currently accepted medical use in treatment in the United States.

- Abuse may lead to limited physical or psychological dependence relative to the drugs or other substances in Schedule III

Included in Schedule IV are the following drugs or substances:

- Narcotic drugs. Unless specifically excepted or unless listed in another schedule, any material, compound, mixture, or preparation containing any of the following narcotic drugs, or their salts calculated as the free an-hydrous base or alkaloid, in limited quantities as set forth below:

  (1) Not more than 1 milligram of difenoxin and not less than 25 micrograms of atropine sulfate per dosage unit

  (2) Dextropropoxyphene (alpha-(+)-4-dimethylamino-1,2-diphenyl-3-methyl-2-propionoxybutane)

- Depressants. Unless specifically excepted or unless listed in another schedule, any material, compound, mixture, or preparation which contains any quantity of the following substances, including its salts, isomers, and salts of isomers:

(1)   Alprazolam
(2)   Barbital
(3)   Bromazepam
(4)   Camazepam
(5)   Chloral betaine
(6)   Chloral hydrate
(7)   Chlordiazepoxide
(8)   Clobazam
(9)   Clonazepam
(10)   Clorazepate
(11)   Clotiazepam
(12)   Cloxazolam
(13)   Delorazepam
(14)   Diazepam
(15)   Dichloralphenazone
(16)   Estazolam
(17)   Ethchlorvynol
(18)   Ethinamate
(19)   Ethyl loflazepate
(20)   Fludiazepam
(21)   Flunitrazepam
(22)   Flurazepam
(23)   Halazepam
(24)   Haloxazolam
(25)   Ketazolam
(26)   Loprazolam
(27)   Lorazepam
(28)   Lormetazepam
(29)   Mebutamate
(30)   Medazepam
(31)   Meprobamate
(32)   Methohexital
(33)   Methylphenobarbital (mephobarbital)
(34)   Midazolam

(35) Nimetazepam
(36) Nitrazepam
(37) Nordiazepam
(38) Oxazepam
(39) Oxazolam
(40) Paraldehyde
(41) Petrichloral
(42) Phenobarbital
(43) Pinazepam
(44) Prazepam
(45) Quazepam
(46) Temazepam
(47) Tetrazepam
(48) Triazolam
(49) Zaleplon
(50) Zolpidem

Study Tip

Note that most of the drugs in the list above are benzodiazepines and end in the suffixes "azolam" or "azepam". Also, important drugs such as phenobarbital, zaleplon and zolpidem are in this category.

- Fenfluramine. Any material, compound, mixture, or preparation which contains any quantity of fenfluramine, including its salts, and salts of such isomers.
- Stimulants. Unless specifically excepted or unless listed in another schedule, any material, compound, mixture, or preparation which contains any quantity of the following substances having a stimulant effect on the central nervous system, including its salts, isomers and salts of isomers:
  (1) Cathine ((+)-norpseudoephedrine)
  (2) Diethylpropion
  (3) Fencamfamin
  (4) Fenproporex

    (5) Mazindol
    (6) Mefenorex
    (7) Modafinil
    (8) Pemoline (including organometallic complexes
         and chelates thereof)
    (9) Phentermine
    (10) Pipradrol
    (11) Sibutramin
    (12) SPA ((-)-1-dimethylamino- 1,2-diphenylethane)

- Other substances. Unless specifically excepted or unless listed in another schedule, any material, compound, mixture or preparation which contains any quantity of the following substances, including its salts:

    (1) Pentazocine
    (2) Butorphanol (including its optical isomers)

Schedule V Controlled Substances

Drugs classified as schedule V controlled substances are those that have the following characteristics:

- Have a low potential for abuse relative to the drugs or other substances in schedule IV
- Have a currently accepted medical use in treatment in the United States
- Abuse of the drug or other substance may lead to limited physical or psychological dependence relative to the drugs or other substances in schedule IV

Schedule V includes the following drugs or substances:

- Buprenorphine

- Narcotic drugs containing non-narcotic active medicinal ingredients. Any compound, mixture, or preparation containing any of the following narcotic drugs, or their salts calculated as the free anhydrous base or alkaloid, in limited quantities as set forth below, which must include one or more non-narcotic active medicinal ingredients in sufficient proportion to confer upon the compound, mixture, or preparation valuable medicinal qualities other than those possessed by narcotic drugs alone:

  (1) Not more than 200 milligrams of codeine per 100 milliliters or per 100 grams.

  (2) Not more than 100 milligrams of dihydrocodeine per 100 milliliters or per 100 grams.

  (3) Not more than 100 milligrams of ethylmorphine per 100 milliliters or per 100 grams.

  (4) Not more than 2.5 milligrams of diphenoxylate and not less than 25 micrograms of atropine sulfate per dosage unit.

  (5) Not more than 100 milligrams of opium per 100 milliliters or per 100 grams.

  (6) Not more than 0.5 milligram of difenoxin and not less than 25 micrograms of atropine sulfate per dosage unit

> ## Study Tip
> Note that all of the quantities listed above are evenly divisible by FIVE. This is a clue that they are classified in Schedule V.

- Stimulants. Unless specifically exempted or excluded or unless listed in another schedule, any material, compound, mixture, or preparation which contains any quantity of pyrovalerone having a stimulant effect on the central nervous system, including its salts, isomers and salts of isomers.

Excluded (Exempt) Substances

The following non-narcotic substances are excluded from all schedules:

Brand Name	Controlled Substance Ingredient
Theophed	Phenobarbital
Guiaphed Elixir	Phenobarbital
Tedrigen Tablets	Phenobarbital
Choate's Leg Freeze	Chloral hydrate
Tedral Tablets	Phenobarbital
Tedral Elixir	Phenobarbital
Tedral S.A Tablets	Phenobarbital
Tedral Suspension	Phenobarbital
Asma-Ese Tablets	Phenobarbital
Azma-Aids Tablets	Phenobarbital
Benzedrex Inhaler	Propylhexedrine
Bronkolixir Elixir	Phenobarbital
Bronkotabs Tablets	Phenobarbital
Vicks Inhaler	l-Desoxyephedrine
Primatene Tablets	Phenobarbital

> ## Note
> Manufacturers may apply to the DEA for exemption of a product from controlled substance status. The exemption may be granted if it appears unlikely that the product can be abused.

Purchasing or Transferring Schedule I or II Substances

An order form (DEA Form 222) is required for each sale or transfer of a schedule I or II controlled substance.

> ## Note
> DEA Form 222 is required for purchases, transfer of schedule I and II products from one pharmacy to another, returns to a supplier, etc.

Order forms may be obtained only by persons who are registered to handle controlled substances listed in schedules I and II, and by persons who are registered to export such substances. Persons not registered to handle controlled substances listed in schedule I or II and persons registered only to import controlled substances listed in any schedule are not entitled to obtain order forms.

An order form may be executed only on behalf of the registrant and only if his/her controlled substance registration has not expired or been revoked or suspended.

When an individual applies for a registration, the applicant may indicate on the application form that order forms are needed.

Order Forms (DEA Form 222) are issued in mailing envelopes containing either seven or fourteen forms, each form containing an original, a duplicate, and a triplicate copy (i.e., Copy 1, Copy 2, and Copy 3) (see Figure I).

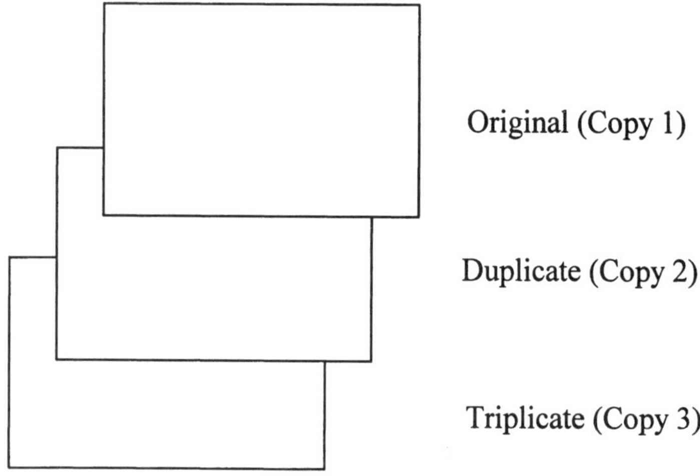

Figure I - Parts of DEA Form 222

A limit, which is based on the business activity of the registrant, is imposed on the number of order forms that are furnished on any requisition unless additional forms are specifically requested and a reasonable need for such additional forms is shown. Additional forms may be requisitioned on the DEA Form 222a that is mailed to a registrant approximately 30 days after each shipment of order forms to that registrant. Registrants may also order additional forms by contacting any Division Office or the Registration Unit of the DEA.

All requisition forms (DEA Form 222a) must be submitted to the Registration Unit of the DEA. Each requisition must show the name, address, and registration number of the registrant and the number of books of order forms desired. Each requisition must be signed and dated by the same person who signed the most recent application for registration or for re-registration or by any person authorized to obtain and execute order forms by a Power of Attorney.

Order forms are serially numbered and issued with the name, address and registration number of the registrant, the authorized activity and schedules of the registrant. This information cannot be altered or changed by the registrant; the Registration Unit of the DEA must correct any errors by returning the forms with notification of the error.

Completing DEA Form 222

Order forms must be prepared and executed by the purchaser simultaneously in triplicate by means of interleaved carbon sheets that are part of the DEA Form 222 (see above). Order forms must be prepared by use of a typewriter, pen, or indelible pencil.

Only one item may be entered on each numbered line of the order form. An item consists of one or more commercial or bulk containers of the same finished or bulk form and quantity of the same substance. The number of lines completed must be noted on that form at the bottom of the form, in the space provided. Order forms for car-fentanil, etorphine hydrochloride, and diprenorphine must contain only these substances.

Note

Remember that when ordering controlled substances on a DEA Form 222, a registrant is not permitted to order different drug products on the SAME LINE. For example, 3 x 100 Percodan tablets may be ordered on one line but not 1 x 100 Percodan and 1 x 100 codeine sulfate 30 mg tablets. Each different product must be ordered on a separate line.

The name and address of the supplier from whom the controlled substances are being ordered must be entered on the form. Only one supplier may be listed on any form.

Each order form must be signed and dated by a person authorized to sign an application for registration. The name of the purchaser, if different from the individual signing the order form, must also be inserted in the signature space.

Unexecuted order forms may be kept and may be executed at a location other than the registered location printed on the form. However, all unused forms must be promptly delivered to the registered site when any federal, state, or local inspector authorized to examine controlled substances, inspects the site.

Any purchaser may authorize one or more individuals to obtain and execute order forms on his/her behalf by creating a Power of Attorney for each such individual. The Power of Attorney must be signed by the same person who signed the most recent application for registration or re-registration and by the individual being given authorization to obtain and execute order forms. The Power of Attorney must be filed with the executed order forms of the purchaser, and must be retained for the same period as any order form bearing the signature of the Attorney. The Power of Attorney must be available for inspection together with other order form records.

Any Power of Attorney may be revoked at any time by executing a Notice of Revocation. This must be signed by the person who signed (or was authorized to sign) the Power of Attorney or by a successor, whoever signed the most recent application for registration or re-registration. It must be filed with the Power of Attorney being revoked. An example of the Power of Attorney form and notice of revocation is provided on the next page.

Filling Orders Written on DEA Form 222

Only a person registered as a manufacturer or distributor of controlled substances listed in Schedule I or II may fill an order form, except for the following:

- A pharmacist who is discontinuing a pharmacy
- If a registrant's registration is expiring without re-registration.
- If a registrant is returning a Schedule I or II substance to the supplier (i.e. wholesaler or manufacturer) from which it was obtained.
- A person registered or authorized to conduct chemical analysis or research with controlled substances may distribute a controlled substance listed in Schedule I or II to another person registered or authorized to do the same.

Power of Attorney for DEA Order Forms

_______________________________(Name of registrant)
_______________________________ (Address of registrant)
_______________________________ (DEA registration number)

I, _____________________ (name of person granting power), the undersigned, who is authorized to sign the current application for registration of the above-named registrant under the Controlled Substances Act or Controlled Substances Import and Export Act, have made, constituted, and appointed, and by these presents, do make, constitute, and appoint _____________________________ (name of attorney-in-fact), my true and lawful attorney for me in my name, place, and stead, to execute applications for books of official order forms and to sign such order forms in requisition for Schedule I and II controlled substances, in accordance with section 308 of the Controlled Substances Act (21 U.S.C. 828) and part 1305 of Title 21 of the Code of Federal Regulations. I hereby ratify and confirm all that said attorney shall lawfully do or cause to be done by virtue hereof ___________________(Signature of person granting power)

I, ________ (name of attorney-in-fact), hereby affirm that I am the person named herein as attorney-in-fact and that the signature affixed hereto is my signature.
_______________________________(Signature of attorney-in-fact)

Witnesses:
1._____________________. 2._____________________.
Signed and dated on the _______ day of __________, (year), at
_______________________.

The foregoing power of attorney is hereby revoked by the undersigned, who is authorized to sign the current application for registration of the above-named registrant under the Controlled Substances Act of the Controlled Substances Import and Export Act. Written notice of this revocation has been given to the attorney-in-fact __________ this same day.

_______________________(Signature of person revoking power)
Witnesses: 1._____________________   2._____________________
Signed and dated on the ________ day of __________, (year), at
__________.

- A person registered as a compounder of narcotic substances for use at off-site locations in conjunction with a narcotic treatment program at the compounding location. Such persons may fill orders for narcotic drugs for off-site narcotic treatment programs only.

Note

In summary, any transfer of Schedule I or II drugs from one registrant to another (e.g. pharmacy to pharmacy, pharmacy to wholesaler or manufacturer, etc.) requires the use of a DEA Form 222.

Ordering Controlled Substances Using DEA Form 222

To order a controlled substance in Schedule I or II the purchaser completes DEA Form 222, submits Copy 1 and Copy 2 of the form to the supplier, and retains Copy 3 in his/her own files. The supplier fills the order, and records on Copies 1 and 2 the number of commercial or bulk containers furnished on each item and the date on which such containers are shipped to the purchaser.

If an order cannot be completely filled, it may be partially filled and the balance supplied by additional shipments within 60 days following the date of the order form. The order form is no longer valid after 60 days from the time it was executed by the purchaser.

The controlled substances may only be shipped to the purchaser and to the location printed by the DEA on the order form.

The supplier must retain Copy 1 of the order form for his/her own files and forward Copy 2, at the close of the month during which the order is filled, to the Special Agent in Charge of the DEA office in the area in which the supplier is located.

Study Tip

The person who fills a controlled substance order always keeps the original portion of the order. In this case, the supplier is "filling" the order for the purchaser. When a prescription is filled, the pharmacist is the supplier and therefore keeps the original prescription.

If a single order is filled by partial shipments, Copy 2 must be forwarded to the regional DEA office at the close of the month during which the final shipment is made or during which the 60-day validity period expires.

The purchaser (i.e. the pharmacist, physician, etc.) must record on Copy 3 of the order form the number of commercial or bulk containers received on each item and the dates on which such containers are received.

Endorsing an Order Form

An order form made out to any supplier who cannot fill all or a part of the order within the specified time limitation may be endorsed to another supplier for filling.

The endorsement must be made only by the supplier to whom the order form was first made and must

- state (in the spaces provided on the reverse sides of Copies 1 and 2 of the order form) the name and address of the second supplier

- be signed by a person authorized to obtain and execute order forms on behalf of the first supplier.

The first supplier may not fill any part of an order on an endorsed form.

The second supplier must fill the order, if possible, and ship all substances directly to the purchaser.

Distributions made on endorsed order forms must be reported by the second supplier in the same manner as all other distributions except that where the name of the supplier is requested on the reporting form, the second supplier must record the name, address and registration number of the first supplier.

Unaccepted or Defective Order Forms

An order form must not be filled if it:

- is not complete, legible, or properly prepared, executed, or endorsed; or

- shows any alteration, erasure, or change of any description.

If an order cannot be filled for any reason, the supplier must return Copies 1 and 2 to the purchaser with a statement as to the reason (e.g., illegible or altered).

A supplier may for any reason refuse to accept any order. If a supplier refuses to accept the order, a statement that the order is not accepted is sufficient. When received by the purchaser, Copies 1 and 2 of the order form and the statement indicating why it was not filled must be attached to Copy 3 and retained in the files of the purchaser.

An order form that is incorrect may not be corrected; in order for the order to be filled, a new order form must replace it.

Lost or Stolen Order Forms

If a purchaser determines that an unfilled order form has been lost, he/she must prepare another form in triplicate. He/she must also prepare a statement containing the serial number and date of the lost form. The statement should indicate that the goods covered by the first order form were not received because that order form was lost.

Copy 3 of the second form and a copy of the statement must be retained with Copy 3 of the order form first executed. A copy of the statement must be attached to Copies 1 and 2 of the second order form sent to the supplier. If the first order form is subsequently received by the supplier to whom it was directed, the supplier must write ``Not accepted" on the face of the form and return Copies 1 and 2 to the purchaser, who must attach it to Copy 3 and the statement.

Whenever any used or unused order forms are stolen or lost (other than in the course of transmission) by any purchaser or supplier, he/she must immediately report the loss to the Special Agent in Charge of the DEA in the Divisional Office responsible for the area in which the registrant is located. The report must state the serial number of each form stolen or lost. If the theft or loss includes any original order forms received from purchasers and the supplier is unable to state the serial numbers of such order forms, he/she must report the date or approximate date of receipt thereof and the names and addresses of the purchasers.

If an entire book of order forms is lost or stolen, and the purchaser is unable to state the serial numbers of the lost order forms, he/she must report the date or approximate date of issuance of the forms instead. If any unused order form reported stolen or lost is subsequently recovered or found, the Special Agent in Charge of the DEA in the Divisional Office responsible for the area in which the registrant is located must immediately be notified.

Study Tip

Carefully review the process of ordering Schedule I and II drugs. An excellent way to review this process is to prepare a simulated, triplicate DEA Form 222 and practice the ordering process, perhaps using a friend as the "supplier".

Storage of Order Forms

The PURCHASER must retain Copy 3 of each order form that has been filled. He/she must also retain in his files all copies of each unaccepted or defective order form and each statement attached thereto. Order forms must be maintained separately from all other records of the Registrant.

The SUPPLIER must retain Copy 1 of each order form that he/she has filled.

Order forms and other related documents must be kept available for inspection for a period of two years.

A supplier of carfentanil, etorphine hydrochloride and diprenorphine must maintain order forms for these substances separately from all other order forms and records.

Note

Carfentanil, etorphine hydrochloride and diprenorphine are potent narcotics that are used exclusively in veterinary practice. They are often used to immobilize large animals.

Return of Unused Order Forms

If the registration of any purchaser terminates (because the purchaser dies, ceases legal existence, discontinues business or professional practice), or changes the name or address as shown on his registration, or if his/her registration is suspended or revoked, all unused order forms must be returned to the nearest office of the DEA.

Cancellation and Voiding of Order Forms

A purchaser may cancel part or all of an order on an order form by notifying the supplier in writing of such cancellation. The supplier must indicate the cancellation on Copies 1 and 2 of the order form by drawing a line through the canceled items and printing "cancelled" in the space provided for number of items shipped.

A supplier may void part or all of an order on an order form by notifying the purchaser in writing of such voiding. The supplier must indicate the voiding in the manner prescribed for cancellation in the previous paragraph.

Persons Entitled To Issue Prescriptions

A prescription for a controlled substance may be issued only by an individual practitioner who is:

- authorized to prescribe controlled substances by the jurisdiction in which he/she is licensed to practice his profession, and

- either registered or exempted from registration pursuant to the CSA.

An employee or agent of the individual practitioner (e.g. a nurse, secretary) may communicate a prescription issued by an individual practitioner to a pharmacist.

Purpose of Issue of Controlled Substances Prescriptions

To be valid, a prescription for a controlled substance must be issued for a legitimate medical purpose by an individual practitioner acting in the usual course of his/her professional practice.

The responsibility for the proper prescribing and dispensing of controlled substances is upon the prescribing practitioner, but a corresponding responsibility rests with the pharmacist who fills the prescription.

An order/prescription that is not issued in the usual course of professional treatment or as part of legitimate and authorized research is not a prescription. A person knowingly filling such an order or prescription, as well as the person issuing it, is in violation of the CSA.

A prescription may not be issued in order for an individual practitioner to obtain controlled substances for the purpose of general dispensing to patients.

Note

If a practitioner wishes to dispense controlled substances to patients, he/she must order them directly from a supplier (i.e. a wholesaler or manufacturer). In other words, prescribing controlled substances for "office use" is not permissible.

A prescription may not be issued for the dispensing of narcotic drugs listed in any schedule for "detoxification treatment" or ``maintenance treatment".

Issuing Of Controlled Substance Prescriptions

All prescriptions for controlled substances must be dated and signed on the day when written and must bear:

- the full name and address of the patient
- the drug name, strength, dosage form
- quantity prescribed
- directions for use
- the name, address and registration number (i.e. DEA number) of the practitioner

A practitioner must sign a prescription in the same manner as he/she would sign a check or legal document (e.g., J.H. Smith or John H. Smith).

Each written prescription must be written in ink or indelible (i.e. not erasable) pencil or typewriter and the practitioner must manually sign it.

An agent of the practitioner (e.g. a secretary or nurse) may prepare prescriptions for the practitioner's signature, but the prescribing practitioner is still responsible for assuring that the prescription conforms in all essential respects to the law and regulations. A corresponding liability rests upon the pharmacist who fills a prescription that is not prepared in proper form.

An individual practitioner exempted from registration under the CSA must instead include on all prescriptions issued by him or her, the registration number of the hospital or other institution and the special internal code number assigned to him or her by the hospital or other institution.

> ## Note
> Many states permit institutions such as hospitals to provide prescribers in the institution who do not have their own registration number with the hospital DEA number plus a numerical suffix that specifically identifies the prescriber.

Each written prescription must have the name of the physician stamped, typed, or hand-printed on it, as well as the signature of the physician.

An official exempted from registration under the CSA (e.g. a military or Public Health Service physician) must include his/her branch of service or agency (e.g., "U.S. Army" or ``Public Health Service") and service identification number on all prescriptions issued, instead of the DEA number usually required. The service identification number for a Public Health Service employee is his/her Social Security number. Each prescription must have the name of the officer stamped, typed, or hand-printed on it, as well as the signature of the officer.

Persons Entitled To Fill Controlled Substance Prescriptions

Only a pharmacist, acting in the usual course of his/her professional practice, may fill a prescription for controlled substances. Such a pharmacist must either be registered individually or employed in a registered pharmacy or registered institutional pharmacy.

Detoxification or Maintenance Treatment

In order to administer or dispense (but not prescribe) narcotic drugs listed in any schedule to a narcotic drug-dependent person for "detoxification treatment" or "maintenance treatment" a practitioner must be separately registered with DEA and must comply with the special regulatory standards imposed relative to treatment qualification, security, records and unsupervised use of drugs.

A physician who is not specifically registered to conduct a narcotic treatment program may administer (but not prescribe) narcotic drugs to a person for the purpose of relieving acute withdrawal symptoms, when necessary, while arrangements are being made for referral for treatment. Not more than one day's medication may be administered to the person or for the person's use at one time. Such emergency treatment may be carried out for not more than three days and may not be renewed or extended.

Schedule II Prescription Requirements

Written Prescriptions and Orders - A pharmacist may normally dispense a Schedule II controlled substance prescription drug only pursuant to a written prescription signed by the practitioner.

An individual practitioner may administer or dispense directly a Schedule II controlled substance in the course of his/her professional practice without a prescription.

An institutional pharmacist or other health care practitioner may administer or dispense directly (but not prescribe):

- a Schedule II controlled substance only pursuant to a written prescription signed by the prescribing practitioner or

- an order for Schedule II medication that is to be dispensed for immediate administration to the ultimate user.

Oral Prescriptions or Orders - In an emergency situation, a pharmacist may dispense a Schedule II controlled substance upon receiving the oral authorization of a prescribing practitioner, provided that:

- The quantity prescribed and dispensed is limited to the amount adequate to treat the patient during the emergency period (dispensing beyond the emergency period must be pursuant to a written prescription signed by the prescribing practitioner).

- The prescription must be immediately reduced to writing by the pharmacist and must contain all required information except for the signature of the prescriber.

- If the pharmacist does not know the prescriber, he/she must make a reasonable effort to determine that the oral order is legitimate. Such effort(s) may include a call-back to the prescriber using his/her phone number as listed in the telephone directory and/or other good faith efforts to insure his/her identity.

- Within seven (7) days after authorizing an emergency oral prescription, the prescriber must have delivered to the dispensing pharmacist a written prescription for the emergency quantity prescribed. In addition to conforming to the usual requirements for written Schedule II drug prescriptions, this "cover" prescription must have written on its face ``Authorization for Emergency Dispensing," and the date of the oral order. The "cover" prescription may be delivered to the pharmacist in person or by mail. If it is delivered by mail it must be postmarked within the 7-day period. Upon receipt of the "cover" prescription, the dispensing pharmacist is required to attach this prescription to the oral emergency prescription that had earlier been reduced to writing.

The pharmacist is required to notify the nearest DEA office if the prescriber fails to deliver a written prescription to him/her.

What Is An Emergency?

For the purposes of authorizing an oral prescription of a controlled substance listed in Schedule II, the term "emergency situation" means those situations in which the prescriber determines:

- that immediate administration of the controlled substance is necessary for proper treatment of the intended ultimate user; and

- that no appropriate alternative treatment is available, including administration of a drug which is not a schedule II controlled substance; and

- that it is not reasonably possible for the prescriber to provide a written prescription to be presented to the person dispensing the substance, prior to the dispensing.

Faxing of Schedule II Prescriptions

Faxing of a Schedule II prescription to the dispensing pharmacy by the prescriber or the prescriber's agent is permitted for:

- narcotic substances to be compounded for the direct administration to a patient by parenteral intravenous, intramuscular, subcutaneous or intraspinal infusion.

- a resident of a Long Term Care Facility (LTCF).

- a patient residing in a hospice certified by or licensed by the state. The practitioner or the practitioner's agent must note on the prescription that the patient is a hospice patient.

In each case, the fax serves as the original written prescription and must be filed accordingly.

Refilling Schedule II Prescriptions

The refilling of Schedule II prescriptions is prohibited.

Partial Filling of Schedule II Prescriptions

The partial filling of Schedule II controlled substance prescriptions is permissible. If the pharmacist is unable to supply the full quantity called for in a written or emergency oral prescription, he/she must make a notation of the quantity supplied on the face of the written prescription (or written record of the emergency oral prescription). The remaining portion of the prescription may be filled within 72 hours of the first partial filling. If the remaining portion is not or cannot be filled within the 72-hour period, the pharmacist must notify the prescribing individual practitioner. No further quantity may be supplied beyond 72 hours without a new prescription.

<table>
<tr><td>

Note

Partial filling of a Schedule II prescription is not permitted if it is being done on the request of the patient (e.g. if a patient only wants half of the medication the prescription calls for). Partial filling is only permitted if the pharmacist is unable to supply the full quantity prescribed (e.g. because he/she is out of stock).

</td></tr>
</table>

A prescription for a Schedule II controlled substance written for a patient in a Long Term Care Facility (LTCF) or for a patient with a medical diagnosis documenting a terminal illness may be filled in partial quantities. If there is any question whether a patient may be classified as having a terminal illness, the pharmacist must contact the prescriber prior to partially filling the prescription. Both the pharmacist and the prescriber have a corresponding responsibility to assure that the controlled substance is for a terminally ill patient. The pharmacist must record on the prescription whether the patient is "terminally ill" or an "LTCF patient'.' A prescription that is partially filled and does not contain the notation "terminally ill" or "LTCF patient" is assumed to have been filled in violation of the CSA.

For each partial filling, the dispensing pharmacist must record on the BACK of the prescription (or on another appropriate record, uniformly maintained, and readily retrievable) the

- date of the partial filling
- quantity dispensed
- remaining quantity authorized to be dispensed
- identification of the dispensing pharmacist

The total quantity of Schedule II controlled substances dispensed in all partial fillings is not permitted to exceed the total quantity prescribed.

Schedule II prescriptions for patients in a LTCF or patients with a medical diagnosis documenting a terminal illness are valid for a period not to exceed 60 days from the issue date.

Information related to current Schedule II prescriptions for patients in a LTCF or for patients with a medical diagnosis documenting a terminal illness may be maintained in a computerized system if this system has the capability to permit:

- output (display or printout) of the original prescription number, date of issue, identification of prescribing individual practitioner, identification of patient, address of the LTCF or address of the hospital or residence of the patient, identification of medication authorized (to include dosage, form, strength and quantity), listing of the partial fillings that have been dispensed under each prescription and other information required by the CSA.

- immediate (real time) updating of the prescription record each time a partial filling of the prescription is conducted.

Labeling Schedule II Prescriptions

The pharmacist filling a written or emergency oral prescription for a Schedule II controlled substance must affix to the prescription package a label showing the

- date of filling
- pharmacy name and address
- serial number of the prescription
- name of the patient
- name of the prescribing practitioner
- directions for use
- following warning: "Caution: Federal law prohibits the transfer of this drug to any person other than the patient for whom it was prescribed."

Note
This "Caution" statement is not required to appear on the label of a Schedule II controlled substance dispensed for use in clinical investigations which are "blinded" (e.g. a double-blinded study).

- other cautionary statements, if any, contained in such prescription or required by law.

These requirements do not apply when a controlled substance listed in Schedule II is prescribed for administration to a patient in an institution, provided that:

- not more than 7-day supply of the Schedule II controlled substance is dispensed at one time.

- the controlled substance listed in Schedule II is not in the possession of the ultimate user prior to the administration.

- the institution maintains appropriate safeguards and records regarding the proper administration, control, dispensing, and storage of the controlled substance listed in Schedule II, and

- The system employed by the pharmacist in filling a prescription is adequate to identify the supplier, the product, and the patient, and to set forth the directions for use and cautionary statements, if any, contained in the prescription or required by law.

Schedule III, IV, and V Prescription Requirements

A pharmacist may dispense a Schedule III, IV, or V controlled substance prescription drug only pursuant to

- a written prescription signed by a practitioner, or

- a fax of a written, signed prescription transmitted by the prescriber or the prescriber's agent to the pharmacy, or

- pursuant to an oral prescription made by an individual practitioner and promptly reduced to writing by the pharmacist containing all information required except for the signature of the prescriber.

A prescriber may administer or dispense a Schedule III, IV, or V controlled substance directly to a consumer in the course of his/her professional practice without a prescription.

An institutional practitioner-pharmacist may administer or dispense directly (but not prescribe) a Schedule III, IV, or V controlled substance only pursuant to

- a written prescription signed by a prescriber.

- a fax of a written prescription or order for medication transmitted by the prescriber or the prescriber's agent to the institutional practitioner-pharmacist.

- an oral prescription made by a prescriber and promptly reduced to writing by the pharmacist (containing all required information except for the signature of the prescriber).

- an order for medication made by a prescriber which is dispensed for immediate administration to the ultimate user.

Refilling of Schedule III, IV or V Prescriptions

Prescriptions for Schedule III or IV controlled substances may be refilled not more than five times in a six month period from the date on which such prescription was issued, if authorized by the prescriber.

A record of each refilling of a prescription must be entered on the back of the prescription or on another appropriate document. If entered on another document, such as a medication record, the document must be uniformly maintained and readily retrievable. The following information must be retrievable by the prescription number:

- name and dosage form of the controlled substance
- date filled or refilled
- quantity dispensed
- initials of the dispensing pharmacist for each refill
- the total number of refills for that prescription

If the pharmacist just initials and dates the back of the prescription it is assumed that the full face amount of the prescription has been dispensed as a refill.

The prescribing practitioner may authorize additional refills of Schedule III or IV controlled substances on the original prescription through an oral refill authorization transmitted to the pharmacist provided the following conditions are met:

- The total quantity authorized, including the amount of the original prescription, does not exceed five refills within a six-month period from the date of issue of the original prescription.

- The pharmacist obtaining the oral authorization must record on the reverse of the original prescription the

    - date of authorization
    - quantity of medication per refill
    - number of additional refills authorized
    - initials of the pharmacist who received the authorization from the prescriber who issued the original prescription.

- The quantity of each additional refill authorized is equal to or less than the quantity authorized for the initial filling of the original prescription.

- The prescriber must issue a new and separate prescription for any additional quantities beyond the five refill, six-month limitation.

As an alternative to the procedures described above, an automated data processing system (i.e. a computer) may be used for the storage and retrieval of refill information for prescription orders for Schedule III and IV controlled substances, subject to the following conditions:

- The computerized system must provide on-line retrieval (via CRT display or hard-copy printout) of original prescription order information for those prescription orders which are currently authorized for refilling. This must include, but is not limited to the:

  - original prescription number
  - date of issuance of the original prescription order by the prescriber
  - full name and address of the patient
  - name, address, and DEA registration number of the prescriber
  - name, strength, dosage form and quantity of the controlled substance prescribed (and quantity dispensed if different from the quantity prescribed)
  - total number of refills authorized by the prescriber

- The computerized system must provide on-line retrieval (via CRT display or hard-copy printout) of the current refill history for Schedule III or IV controlled substance prescription orders (those authorized for refill during the past six months.) This refill history must include, but is not limited to the

- name of the controlled substance
- date of refill
- quantity dispensed
- identification code, or name or initials of the dispensing pharmacist for each refill
- total number of refills dispensed to date for that prescription order.

• Documentation of the fact that the refill information entered into the computer each time a pharmacist refills an original prescription order for a Schedule III or IV controlled substance is correct must be provided by the individual pharmacist who makes use of such a system.

• If such a system provides a hard-copy printout of each day's controlled substance prescription order refill data, that printout must be verified, dated, and signed by the individual pharmacist who refilled such a prescription order. The individual pharmacist must verify that the data indicated is correct and then sign this document in the same manner as he/she would sign a check or legal document (e.g., C. H. Smith, or Chris H. Smith). This document must be maintained in a separate file at that pharmacy for a period of two years from the dispensing date. This printout of the day's controlled substance prescription order refill data must be provided to each pharmacy using such a computerized system within 72 hours of the date on which the refill was dispensed. It must be verified and signed by each pharmacist who is involved with such dispensing. In lieu of such a printout, the pharmacy must maintain a bound log book, or separate file, in which each individual pharmacist involved in such dispensing must sign a statement each day. The statement must attest to the fact that the refill information entered into the computer that day has been reviewed by him/her and is correct as shown. Such a book or file must be maintained at the pharmacy using such a system for a period of two years after the date of dispensing the appropriately authorized refill.

- Any such computerized system must have the capability of producing a printout of any refill data that the user pharmacy is responsible for maintaining under the CSA. For example, this would include a refill-by-refill audit trail for any specified strength and dosage form of any controlled substance (by either brand or generic name or both). Such a printout must include

  - name of the prescriber
  - name and address of the patient
  - quantity dispensed on each refill
  - date of dispensing for each refill
  - name or identification code of the dispensing pharmacist
  - the number of the original prescription order

- In any computerized system employed by a user pharmacy, the central record-keeping location must be capable of sending the printout to the pharmacy within 48 hours.

- In the event that a pharmacy employing such a computerized system experiences system downtime, the pharmacy must have an auxiliary procedure which will be used for documenting refills of Schedule III and IV controlled substance prescription orders. This auxiliary procedure must insure that refills are authorized by the original prescription order, that the maximum number of refills has not been exceeded, and that all of the appropriate data is retained for on-line data entry as soon as the computer system is available for use again.

> ## Note
> When filing refill information for original pre-
> scription orders for Schedule III or IV controlled
> substances, a pharmacy may use only one of the
> two systems described above (i.e. putting the
> information on the back of the original prescrip-
> tion or onto a computerized record-keeping sys-
> tem).

Partial Filling of Schedule III, IV, and V Prescriptions

The partial filling of a prescription for a controlled sub-
stance listed in Schedule III, IV, or V is permissible, pro-
vided that:

- Each partial filling is recorded in the same manner as a refill (see above).

- The total quantity dispensed in all partial fillings does not exceed the total quantity prescribed.

- No dispensing occurs beyond 6 months after the date on which the prescription was issued.

Labeling and Filling of Schedule III, IV and V Prescriptions

The pharmacist filling a prescription for a Schedule III, IV, or V controlled substance must affix to the package a label showing the

- pharmacy name and address
- serial number
- date of initial filling
- name of the patient
- name of the practitioner issuing the prescription
- directions for use
- the following warning: "Caution: Federal law prohibits the transfer of this drug to any person other than the patient for whom it was prescribed".

Note

This "Caution" statement is NOT required to appear on the label of a controlled substance in Schedule V or for any controlled substance dispensed for use in clinical investigations which are "blinded".

- cautionary statements, if any, contained in the prescripttion, as required by law.

These requirements do not apply when a Schedule III, IV, or V controlled substance is prescribed for administration to an ultimate user who is institutionalized, provided that:

- not more than a 34-day supply or 100 dosage units, whichever is less, of the controlled substance listed in Schedule III, IV, or V is dispensed at one time.

- the controlled substance listed in Schedule III, IV, or V is not in the possession of the ultimate user prior to administration.

- the institution maintains appropriate safeguards and records the proper administration, control, dispensing, and storage of the Schedule III, IV, or V controlled substances.

- the system employed by the pharmacist in filling a prescription is adequate to identify the supplier, the product and the patient, and to include the directions for use and cautionary statements, if any, contained in the prescription or required by law.

Transfer of Prescription Information Between Pharmacies

Original prescription information for a Schedule III, IV or V controlled substance may be transferred on a one-time basis only for the purpose of refill dispensing.

Pharmacies electronically sharing a real-time, on-line database may transfer up to the maximum refills permitted by law and the prescriber's authorization.

All transfers of Schedule III, IV or V controlled substance prescription information are subject to the following requirements:

- The transfer is communicated directly between two licensed pharmacists and the transferring pharmacist enters the following information:

  - Writes the word ``VOID'' on the face of the invalidated prescription.

  - Records on the reverse side of the invalidated prescription the name, address and DEA registration number of the pharmacy to which it was transferred and the name of the pharmacist receiving the prescription information.

  - Records the date of the transfer and the name of the pharmacist transferring the information.

- The pharmacist receiving the transferred prescription information must record in writing the following:

  - Writes the word "transfer" on the face of the transferred prescription.

  - Enters all information required on a prescription by the CSA including the:

    * date of issuance of original prescription

    * original number of refills authorized on the original prescription

    * date of original dispensing

    * number of valid refills remaining

    * date(s) and locations of previous refill(s)

    * pharmacy's name, address, DEA registration number and prescription number from which

       the prescription information was transferred

  * name of pharmacist who transferred the prescription

  * pharmacy's name, address, DEA registration number and prescription number from which the prescription was originally filled

- The original and transferred prescription(s) must be maintained for a period of two years from the date of last refill.

Pharmacies electronically accessing the same prescription record must satisfy all information requirements as for the transfer of manual prescriptions.

The procedure allowing the transfer of prescription information for refill purposes is permissible only if allowable under existing state or other applicable law.

Dispensing Controlled Substances Without a Prescription

A Schedule II, III, IV, or V controlled substance that is not a prescription drug pursuant to any federal, state or local law may be dispensed by a pharmacist without a prescription to a retail purchaser provided that:

- such dispensing is made only by a pharmacist, and not by a non-pharmacist employee even if under the supervision of a pharmacist (although after the pharmacist has fulfilled his/her professional and legal responsibilities, the actual cash, credit transaction, or delivery, may be completed by a non-pharmacist)

> ## Note
> Only a pharmacist may dispense an OTC controlled substance, although a non-pharmacist may complete the sale.

- not more than 240mL (8 ounces) of any such controlled substance containing opium, nor more than 120 mL (4 fluid ounces) of any other such controlled substance nor more than 48 dosage units of any such controlled substance containing opium, nor more than 24 dosage units of any other such controlled substance may be dispensed at retail to the same purchaser in any given 48-hour period.

> ## Note
> Therefore, a pharmacist who sells a codeine-containing cough preparation over-the-counter may not sell more than 4 fluid ounces to a given purchaser in any 48-hour period.

- the purchaser is at least 18 years of age.

- the pharmacist must require every purchaser of a controlled substance not known to him/her to furnish suitable identification (including proof of age where appropriate).

- a bound record book for dispensing controlled substances without a prescription must be maintained by the pharmacist. The book must contain the

  - name and address of each purchaser

- name and quantity of controlled substance purchased

- date of each purchase

- name or initials of the pharmacist who dispensed the substance to the purchaser

The record book must be maintained as other records described in the CSA.

Destruction of Controlled Substances

Once each calendar year retail pharmacies may request DEA authorization to destroy damaged, outdated or otherwise unwanted controlled substances. The pharmacy must complete DEA Form 41 (Registrant's Inventory of Drugs Surrendered), listing all drugs to be destroyed. In addition, the pharmacy must prepare a letter requesting permission to destroy the controlled substances, proposing a date and method of destruction, and listing the names of at least two people who will witness the destruction. The witnesses should be a licensed physician, pharmacist, mid-level practitioner, nurse, or a state or local law enforcement officer. Both documents must be received by the nearest DEA Diversion Field Office at least two weeks prior to the proposed destruction date.

After reviewing all available information, the DEA office will then notify the registrant in writing of its decision. Once the controlled substances have been destroyed, signed copies of the DEA Form 41 must be forwarded to DEA. The pharmacist should contact local environmental authorities prior to implementing the proposed method of destruction to ascertain that there are no hazards associated with the destruction.

A pharmacy may at any time forward controlled substances to DEA registered distributors who handle the disposal of drugs. The pharmacist may contact their local DEA Diversion Field Office for an updated list of those distributors in their area. When a pharmacy transfers Schedule II substances to a distributor for destruction, the distributor must issue an Official Order Form (DEA Form-222) to the pharmacy. When Schedule III-V controlled substances are transferred to a distributor for destruction, the pharmacy should document in writing the drug name, dosage form, strength, quantity and date transferred.

The DEA registered distributor who will destroy the controlled substances is responsible for submitting a DEA Form 41 to DEA when the drugs have been destroyed. A DEA Form 41 should not be used to record the transfer of controlled substances between the pharmacy and the registered distributor disposing the drugs. Prior DEA authorization to destroy controlled substances is not necessary when an authorized member of a state law enforcement authority or regulatory agency witnesses the destruction. Copies of a DEA Form 41 or state controlled substance destruction form must be forwarded to the local DEA Diversion Office after the destruction.

DEA will issue a "Blanket Authorization" for destruction of controlled substances on a very limited basis to those registrants who are associated with hospitals, clinics or other registrants having to dispose of used needles, syringes or other injectable objects only. This limited exception is granted because of the probability that those objects have been contaminated by hazardous bodily fluids. DEA will evaluate requests for a blanket authorization based on the following guidelines:

- Frequency of destruction (i.e., daily, weekly) and volume of drugs involved that warrant such authorization.

- Method of destruction. Drugs must be destroyed in such a manner that they are beyond reclamation (e.g.incineration).

- Registrant's past history.

- Security at the pharmacy or registered location.

- Name and position of the individual responsible for the destruction.

Those registrants granted blanket authorization to destroy controlled substances must complete DEA Form 41.

Note

A pharmacist who wishes to dispose of a controlled substance must, therefore, complete and submit DEA Form 41 to the local DEA Special Agent in Charge at least two weeks prior to the intended disposal. The Form must list those substances which are to be destroyed. The Special Agent will then determine and direct the pharmacist as to how to go about disposing of the substance(s). Such prior authorization is not required if an authorized member of a state law enforcement authority or regulatory agency witnesses the destruction.

Transfer of Controlled Substances Between Pharmacies

A pharmacy practitioner who is registered to dispense controlled substances may distribute (without being registered to distribute) a quantity of such substance to another pharmacy practitioner for the purpose of general dispensing to his/her patients, provided that

- the practitioner to whom the controlled substance is to be distributed is registered under the Con-trolled Substances Act to dispense that controlled substance;

- fhe distribution is recorded by the distributing practitioner and by the receiving practitioner;

- if the substance is listed in Schedule I or II, an order form (DEA Form 222) is used;

- the total number of dosage units of all controlled substances distributed by the practitioner during each calendar year in which the practitioner is registered to dispense does not exceed five percent of the total number of dosage units of all controlled substances distributed and dispensed by the practitioner during the same calendar year;

- If, during any calendar year in which the pharmacy practitioner is registered to dispense, he/she has reason to believe that the total number of dosage units of all controlled substances which will be distributed by him/her will exceed 5 percent of the total number of dosage units of all controlled substances distributed and dispensed by him/her during that calendar year, the practitioner must obtain a registration to distribute controlled substances.

Note

In other words, a pharmacist may transfer up to 5% of the total dosage units of controlled substances dispensed in a given calendar year by the pharmacy without getting wholesaler's permit. DEA Form 222 must also be used in transferring Schedule I and/or II controlled substances to another pharmacy.

If a pharmacy goes out of business or is acquired by a new pharmacy, it may transfer the controlled substances to another pharmacy, supplier, manufacturer or distributor registered to dispose of controlled substances.

To transfer Schedule II substances, the receiving registrant must issue an Official Order Form (DEA Form 222) to the registrant transferring the drugs.

The transfer of Schedule III-V controlled substances must be documented in writing to show the drug name, dosage form, strength, quantity and date transferred. The document must include the names, addresses and DEA registration numbers of the parties involved in the transfer of the controlled substances.

If a pharmacy going out of business wishes to transfer its controlled substances to another pharmacy, the pharmacy must, on the day the controlled substances are transferred, take a complete inventory, which documents the drugs' name, dosage form, strength, quantity, and date transferred. In addition, a DEA Form 222 must be prepared to document the transfer of Schedule II controlled substances. This inventory will serve as the final inventory for the registrant going out of business and transferring the controlled substances. It will also serve as the initial inventory for the registrant acquiring the controlled substances. A copy of the inventory must be included in the records of each person. It is not necessary to send a copy of the inventory to the DEA. The person acquiring the controlled substances must maintain all records involved in the transfer of the controlled substances for two years.

Controlled Substance Records

Prescribers

Prescribers are required to keep records of controlled substances in schedules II, III, IV, and V that are dispensed, other than by prescribing or administering, in their practice. Such practitioners are NOT required to keep records of controlled substances in schedules II, III, IV, and V which are prescribed in the lawful course of their practice, unless such substances are prescribed as part of a maintenance or detoxification treatment of an individual.

Prescribers are not required to keep records of controlled substances listed in Schedules II, III, IV and V that are administered in their practice unless the prescriber regularly engages in the dispensing or administering of controlled substances and charges patients, either separately or together, with charges for other professional services, for substances so dispensed or administered.

Records must be kept for controlled substances administered in the course of maintenance or detoxification treatment of an individual.

Mid-level Practitioners

Each registered mid-level practitioner must maintain, in a readily retrievable manner, those documents required by the state in which he/she practices which describe the conditions and extent of his/her authorization to dispense controlled substances. The practitioner must make such documents available for inspection and copying by authorized employees of the DEA. Examples of such documentation include protocols, practice guidelines or practice agreements.

Pharmacists

Each registered pharmacy must maintain the following inventories and records of controlled substances:

- Inventories and records of all controlled substances listed in Schedules I and II must be maintained separately from all other records of the pharmacy, and prescriptions for such substances must be maintained in a separate prescription file.

- Inventories and records of controlled substances listed in Schedules III, IV, and V must be maintained either separately from all other records of the pharmacy or in such form that the information required is readily retrievable from ordinary business records of the pharmacy. Prescriptions for such substances must be maintained either in a separate prescription file for controlled substances listed in Schedules III, IV, and V only or in such form that they are readily retrievable from the other prescription records of the pharmacy.

- Prescriptions will be deemed readily retrievable if, at the time they are initially filed, the face of the prescription is stamped in red ink in the lower right corner with the letter "C" no less than 1 inch high and filed either in the prescription file for controlled substances listed in Schedules I and II or in the usual consecutively numbered prescription file for non-controlled substances.

- If a pharmacy employs an automatic data processing (computer) system or other electronic record-keeping system for prescriptions which permits identification by prescription number and retrieval of original documents by prescriber's name, patient's name, drug dispensed, and date filled, then the requirement to mark the hard copy prescription with a red "C" is waived.

<table>
<tr><td>

Note

Schedule III, IV, or V prescriptions need NOT be stamped with the red letter "C" if a computer record of these prescriptions is maintained.

</td></tr>
</table>

Other Entities

Each registered manufacturer, distributor, importer, exporter, narcotic treatment program and compounder for narcotic treatment program must maintain the following inventories and records of controlled substances:

- Inventories and records of controlled substances listed in Schedules I and II must be maintained separately from all of the records of the registrant; and

- Inventories and records of controlled substances listed in Schedules III, IV, and V must be maintained either separately from all other records of the registrant or in such form that the information required is readily retrievable from the ordinary business records of the registrant.

Inventory Requirements

Every required inventory and other records must be kept by the registrant and be available, for at least 2 years from the date of such inventory or records, for inspection and copying by authorized employees of the DEA.

Records and inventories of Schedule II controlled substances must be maintained separately from all other records of the registrant. All records and inventories of Schedule III, IV and V controlled substances must be maintained either separately from all other records or in such a form that the information required is readily retrievable from the ordinary business records.

Financial and shipping records (such as invoices and packing slips) may be kept at a central location (e.g. at the main office of a chain pharmacy), rather than at the registered location, if the registrant has notified the DEA of his/her intention to keep central records.

Each controlled substance inventory must contain a complete and accurate record of all controlled substances on hand on the date the inventory is taken, and must be maintained in written, typewritten, or printed form at the registered location. An inventory taken by use of an oral recording device must be promptly transcribed.

Controlled substances must be inventoried if they are in the possession of or under the control of the registrant. These include substances

- returned by a customer
- ordered by a customer but not yet invoiced
- stored in a warehouse on behalf of the registrant
- in the possession of employees of the registrant and intended for distribution as complimentary samples.

A separate inventory must be made for each registered location and each independent activity registered. In the event controlled substances in the possession or under the control of the registrant are stored at a location for which he/she is not registered, the substances must be included in the inventory of the registered location to which they are subject to control or to which the person possessing the substance is responsible.

The inventory may be taken either as of opening of business or as of the close of business on the inventory date and this must be indicated on the inventory.

Every registrant is required to take an inventory of all stocks of controlled substances on hand on the date he/she first engages in the manufacture, distribution, or dispensing of controlled substances. In the event a person commences business with no controlled substances on hand, he/she must record this fact as the initial inventory.

After the initial inventory is taken, the registrant must take a new inventory of all stocks of controlled substances on hand at least every two years. The biennial inventory may be taken on any date that is within two years of the previous biennial inventory date.

Note

A controlled substance inventory must be taken at least once every two years.

When the status of a non-controlled substance is changed to that of a controlled substance, each registrant who possesses that substance must take an inventory of all stocks of the substance on hand. Thereafter, the substance must be included in each inventory made by the registrant.

When conducting a controlled substance inventory, the registrant must make an exact count of substances in sealed, unopened containers. For opened containers the following should be performed:

- If the substance is listed in Schedule I or II, make an exact count or measure of the contents.

- If the substance is listed in Schedule III, IV or V, make an estimated count or measure of the contents, unless the container holds more than 1,000 tablets or capsules in which case an exact count of the contents must be made.

Every registrant must maintain on a current basis a complete and accurate record of each controlled substance manufactured, imported, received, sold, delivered, exported, or otherwise disposed of by him/her. The records must be maintained in a dispensing log at the narcotic treatment program site. No registrant is required to maintain a perpetual inventory.

Each person registered or authorized to maintain and/or detoxify users of controlled substance, as part of a narcotic treatment program, must maintain records with the following information for each narcotic controlled substance:

- Name of substance
- Strength of substance
- Dosage form
- Date dispensed
- Adequate identification of patient (consumer)
- Amount consumed
- Amount and dosage form taken home by patient
- Dispenser's initials

All sites that compound a bulk narcotic solution from bulk narcotic powder to liquid for on-site use must keep a separate batch record of the compounding.

Records of identity, diagnosis, prognosis, or treatment of any patients, which are maintained in connection with the operation of a narcotic treatment program, must be confidential.

Extensive record keeping is required of individuals authorized to compound narcotic drugs for off-site use in a narcotic treatment program.

Verification of DEA Numbers

Knowing how a DEA registration number is constructed can be a useful tool for recognizing a forged prescription. Prior to October 1, 1985, DEA registration numbers for physicians, dentists, veterinarians and other practitioners started with the letter A. Registration numbers issued to practitioners after that date begin with the letter B. Registration numbers issued to mid-level practitioners begin with the letter M. The first letter of the registration number is followed by the first letter of the registrant's last name. (e.g., J for Jones or S for Smith), and then a computer generated sequence of seven numbers (e.g. MJ3614511).

A pharmacist may verify a prescriber's DEA number by performing the following calculation:

Assuming that the DEA number to verify is BR2398328

- Add the 1st, 3rd, and 5th digits of the number
  $2 + 9 + 3 = 14$

- Add the 2nd, 4th, and 6th digits of the number and multiply this sum by 2.
  $3 + 8 + 2 = 13$ $13 \times 2 = 26$

- Add the results of the first two calculations
  $14 + 26 = 40$

The last digit of this final sum (in this case, "0") should be the same as the last digit (i.e. the 7th and final digit) of the DEA number being tested. Since the last digit of the DEA number provided is "8", it is not a valid DEA number. The final number should be "0" to make it a valid number.

Prescribing by Hospital Employees

An individual practitioner (e.g., intern, resident, staff physician, mid-level practitioner) who is an agent or employee of a hospital or other institution may, when acting in the usual course of business or employment, administer, dispense or prescribe controlled substances under the registration of the hospital or other institution in which he or she is employed, provided that the:

- dispensing, administering, or prescribing is in the usual course of his/her professional practice;

- practitioner is authorized to do so by the state in which he or she is practicing;

- hospital or institution has verified that the practitioner is permitted to dispense, administer or prescribe controlled substances within the state;

- practitioner acts only within the scope of his/her employment in the hospital or institution;

- The hospital or institution authorizes the practitioner to dispense or prescribe under its registration and assigns a specific internal code number for each practitioner so authorized (See example of a specific internal code number below);

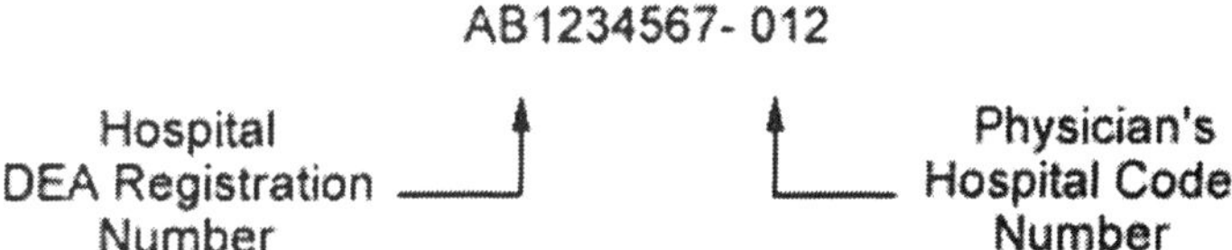

A current list of internal codes and the corresponding individual practitioners should be kept by the hospital or other institution. This list must be available at all times to other registrants and law enforcement agencies upon request for the purpose of verifying the authority of the prescribing individual practitioner. Pharmacists should contact the hospital or other institution for verification if they have any doubts in dispensing such a prescription.

Mid-level Practitioners (MLP)

Mid-level practitioners (MLP) are registered and authorized by the DEA and the state in which they practice to dispense, administer and prescribe controlled substances in the course of their professional practice. Examples of MLPs include, but are not limited to, health care providers such as nurse practitioners, nurse midwives, nurse anesthetists, clinical nurse specialists, physician assistants, optometrists, ambulance services, animal shelters, veterinarian euthanasia technicians, nursing homes and homeopathic physicians.

MLPs may receive an individual DEA registration granting controlled substance privileges. However, such a registration is contingent upon authority granted by the state in which they are licensed. DEA registers MLPs whose states clearly authorize them to prescribe, dispense and administer controlled substances in one or more schedules. The fact that an MLP has been issued a valid DEA registration number (beginning with the letter M) will be evidence that he/she is authorized to prescribe, dispense and/or administer at least some controlled substances. However, it will still be incumbent upon the pharmacist who fills the prescription to ensure that the MLP is prescribing within the parameters established by the state in which he/she practices.

MLP authority to prescribe controlled substances varies greatly by state. Check with your state licensing or controlled substances authority to determine which MLP disciplines are authorized to prescribe controlled substances in your state.

Storage of Controlled Substances

Practitioners and non-practitioners authorized to conduct research or chemical analysis must store controlled substances listed in Schedules II, III, IV, and V in a securely locked, substantially constructed cabinet. However, pharmacies and institutional practitioners may disperse such substances throughout the stock of non-controlled substances in such a manner as to obstruct the theft or diversion of the controlled substances. An electronic alarm system is also recommended.

Carfentanil, etorphine hydrochloride and diprenorphine must be stored in a safe or steel cabinet equivalent to a U.S. Government Class V security container.

Pharmacy Employment Practices

A pharmacy registrant (i.e., the registrant or corporation that owns the pharmacy) must not employ in a position which allows access to controlled substances, anyone who has been convicted of a felony relating to controlled substances, or who, at any time, has had an application for DEA registration denied, revoked, or surrendered for cause. "For cause" means surrendering a registration in lieu of, or as a consequence of, any federal or state administrative, civil or criminal action resulting from an investigation of the individual's handling of controlled substances.

Pharmacies desiring to employ an individual who meets this definition may request an exception to this requirement from the DEA. The employer must have a waiver approved before hiring the applicant. A waiver request should be sent to DEA Headquarters, Office of Diversion Control, Washington, D.C. 20537.

A pharmacy registrant who applies for such a waiver should understand that the following factors will be considered:

- A detailed description of the nature and extent of the applicant's past controlled substances violations.

- Activities of the applicant since the violation.

- Current status of the applicant's state licensure.

- Extent of the applicant's proposed access to controlled substances.

- Registrant's proposed physical and professional safeguards to prevent diversion by the applicant, if employed.

- Status of employing registrant regarding handling of controlled substances.

- Other pertinent information uncovered by DEA in its investigation of the applicant's or registrant's handling of controlled substances.

Such a waiver should not be considered unless there are valid reasons to believe that diversion is unlikely to occur.

Theft of Controlled Substances

Immediately upon discovery of a theft or significant loss of controlled substances, a pharmacy must contact the nearest DEA Diversion Field Office by telephone, facsimile or by a brief written message explaining the circumstances. A pharmacy should also notify the local police as may be required by state law. If there is a question as to whether a theft has occurred or a loss is significant, a registrant should err on the side of caution and report it to DEA.

The DEA must be notified directly. This requirement is not satisfied by reporting the theft or significant loss in any other manner. For example, a corporation which owns/operates multiple registered sites and wishes to channel all notifications through corporate management or any other internal department responsible for security must still provide notice directly to DEA "upon discovery" and keep a copy for its records.

A pharmacy must also complete a DEA Form 106 (Report of Theft or Loss of Controlled Substances). The DEA Form 106 will formally document the actual circumstances of the theft or significant loss and the quantities of controlled substances involved, once this information has been determined conclusively. The pharmacy should send the original DEA Form 106 and a copy to the DEA Diversion Field Office and keep a copy for its records.

When all or part of a shipment disappears, or never reaches its intended destination, the supplier is responsible for reporting the in-transit loss of controlled substances to DEA. A pharmacy is responsible for reporting any loss of controlled substances after a pharmacist has signed for or taken custody of a shipment. If it's discovered after that point that an in-transit loss or theft has occurred, the pharmacist must submit a DEA Form 106.

If, after an investigation of the circumstances surrounding the theft or significant loss it is determined that no such theft or significant loss occurred, no DEA Form 106 need be filed. However, the registrant should notify DEA in writing of this fact in order to resolve the initial report and explain why no DEA Form 106 was filed regarding the incident.

Breakage, damage or spillage does not constitute a "loss of controlled substances". In such situations, any recoverable controlled substances must be disposed of according to DEA requirements, and a DEA Form 41 should be filed.

Federal Investigation of Pharmaceutical Theft or Robbery

The Controlled Substances Registrant Protection Act of 1984 (CSRPA) provides for the federal investigation of pharmaceutical thefts and robberies if any of the following conditions are met:

- Replacement cost of the controlled substances taken is $500 or more.

- A registrant or other person is killed or suffers "significant" bodily injury during the commission of the robbery or theft of a controlled substance.

- Interstate or foreign commerce is involved in planning or executing the crime.

Required Records

The following records must be maintained by a registrant:

- Official Order Forms (DEA Form 222)
- Power of Attorney authorization to sign Order Forms.
- Receipts and invoices for Schedule III, IV, and V controlled substances.
- All inventory records of controlled substances, including the initial and biennial inventories.
- Records of controlled substances distributed or dispensed (i.e., prescriptions).
- Report of Theft or Loss (DEA Form 106).
- Inventory of Drugs Surrendered for Disposal (DEA Form 41).
- Records of transfers of controlled substances between pharmacies.
- DEA registration certificate.

Study Hint

This list provides a great review of documents that you must be familiar with. If you still don't understand the use of each, review previous sections.

Storing Prescription Information

Pharmacies have three options for filing prescription records under the Code of Federal Regulations. If there is a conflict between federal and state requirements for filing prescriptions, DEA recognizes that the pharmacy must choose a filing system that would comply with both federal and state law.

All prescription records must be readily retrievable for DEA inspection. Controlled substance prescriptions must be filed in one of the following three ways:

Option 1 (Three separate files)

- A file for Schedule II drugs dispensed,

- A file for Schedule III, IV and V drugs dispensed, and

- A file for prescription orders for all noncontrolled drugs dispensed.

Option 2 (Two separate files)

- A file for all Schedule II drugs dispensed.

- A file for all other drugs dispensed (noncontrolled and those in Schedule III, IV and V). If this method is used, a prescription for a Schedule III, IV and V drug must be made readily identifiable and retrievable by use of a red "C" stamp not less than one inch high.*

Option 3 (Two separate files)

- A file for all Schedule II-V controlled substances. If this method is used, a prescription for a Schedule III, IV and V drug must be made readily retrievable by use of a red "C" stamp not less than one inch high*.

- A file for prescription orders for all noncontrolled drugs dispensed.

A pharmacy is permitted to use a data processing system as an alternative to the manual method for the storage and retrieval of prescription order refill information for Schedules III, IV and V controlled substances.

The computer system must provide on-line retrieval of original prescription information for those prescriptions which are currently authorized for refill. The information must include, but is not limited to the original prescription number, date of issuance, full name and address of the patient, the prescriber's name, address, and DEA Registration number; the name, strength, dosage form and quantity of the controlled substance prescribed; and the total number of refills authorized by the prescriber.

In addition, the computer system must provide on-line retrieval of the current refill history for Schedule III, IV, or V controlled substance prescriptions. This information must include, but is not limited to the:

* If a pharmacy has an electronic record-keeping system for prescriptions which permits identification by prescription number and retrieval of original documents by prescriber's name, patient's name, drug dispensed and date filled, then the requirements to mark the hard copy prescription with a red "C" is waived.

- name of the controlled substance
- date of refill
- quantity dispensed
- dispensing pharmacist's identification code, or name/initials for each refill
- total number of refills dispensed to date for that prescription.

The pharmacist must verify and document that the refill data entered into the system is correct. All computer generated prescription/refill documentation must be stored in a separate file at the pharmacy and be maintained for a two-year period from the dispensing date.

The pharmacy's computer system must comply with the following guidelines:

- If the system provides a hard copy printout of each day's controlled substance prescription refills, each pharmacist who refilled those prescriptions must verify their accuracy by signing and dating the printout as he/she would sign a check or legal document.

- This printout must be provided to each pharmacy which uses the computer system within 72 hours of the date on which the refill was dispensed. The printout must be verified and signed by each pharmacist who dispensed the refills in the pharmacy.

- In lieu of such a printout, the pharmacy must maintain a bound log book, or separate file in which each pharmacist involved in the day's dispensing signs a statement verifying that the refill information entered into the computer that day has been carefully reviewed by him/her and is correct.

- A pharmacy computer system must have the capability of printing out any refill data which the pharmacy must maintain under the Controlled Substances Act. For example, this would include a refill-by-refill audit trail for any specified strength and dosage form of any controlled substance, by either brand or generic name or both, dispensed by the pharmacy. Such a printout must include the:

  - prescribing practitioner's name.
  - patient's name and address.
  - quantity dispensed on each refill.
  - dispensing date for each refill.
  - name or identification code of the dispensing pharmacist.
  - original prescription number.

In any computerized system employed by a user pharmacy, the central record-keeping location must be capable of providing a printout to a requesting pharmacy of the above information within 48 hours.

In case a pharmacy's computer system experiences downtime, the pharmacy must have a back-up procedure to document in writing refills of Schedule III, IV and V substances. This procedure must ensure that refills are authorized by the original prescription, that the maximum number of refills has not been exceeded, and that all required data is retained for on-line entry as soon as possible.

A pharmacy may use only one of the two systems described (i.e., manual or computer).

Sample Questions

1. A suppository dosage form of amobarbital is likely
    to be classified in which of the following controlled
    substance schedules?
    (A)   I
    (B)   II
    (C)   III
    (D)   IV
    (E)   V

2. DEA Form 222 must be used when which of the
    following classes of controlled substances are
    purchased?
    I.   Schedule III
    II.   Schedule II
    III.   Schedule I
    A. I only   B. III only   C. I & II only
    D. II & II only E. I, II & III

3. Which of the following digits would make the
    following DEA number an authentic one?
                    BC445987__
        (A)   6
        (B)   7
        (C)   8
        (D)   9
        (E)   0

4. A prescriber may authorize a maximum of how
    many refills on a prescription for Percodan tablets?
    (A) 0   (B) 1   (C) 2   (D) 5   (E) 10

5. What percentage of the controlled substance doses dispensed each year may be transferred to another pharmacy without requiring registration as a wholesaler?

(A) 0   (B) 5   (C) 7   (D) 10   (E) 20

6. A partial filling of a Schedule II prescription is permissible under which of the following circumstances?

    I.   The patient is over 65 and only wants half the number of doses prescribed by the physician because he cannot afford the full amount.

    II.   The prescriber indicates that she would like the patient to get half the prescription today and the rest in a week if the medication agrees with him.

    III.   The pharmacist is out of stock and will provide the balance of the prescription to the patient in two days.

A. I only   B. III only   C. I & II only
D. II & III only   E. I, II & III

7. A product that contains not more than 200 mg of codeine per 100 mL of product is classified in controlled substance category:

(A)   noncontrolled
(B)   Schedule II
(C)   Schedule III
(D)   Schedule IV
(E)   Schedule V

8.   When using a DEA Form 222 the center portion of the 3-part form ultimately ends up with the
(A)   purchaser
(B)   state board of pharmacy
(C)   supplier
(D)   regional poison control center
(E)   DEA

9.   Which of the following hospital employees may be permitted to prescribe controlled substances even though they do not have a DEA registration number?
I.   Medical Interns
II.   Medical Residents
III.   Mid-level practitioners
A. I only   B. III only   C. I & II only
D. II & III only   E. I, II & III

10.   Controlled substances may be stored in a pharmacy
I.   in a securely locked cabinet
II.   dispersed through the pharmacy department with non-controlled drug products.
III.   on a controlled substance shelf in the pharmacy department.
A. I only   B. III only   C. I & II only
D. II & III only   D. I, II & III

Answers: 1. C   2. D   3. B   4. A   5. B
           6. B   7. E   8. E   9. E   10. C

Section H

Treatment of Narcotic Dependence

The use of methadone as a way to wean narcotic-dependent individuals from opiates began with the passage of the Comprehensive Drug Abuse Prevention and Control Act of 1970. This approach to treatment has been very controversial because methadone itself is a controlled substance capable of being abused and has at times been diverted into illicit channels. The Narcotic Addict Treatment Act (NATA) of 1974 provided for more stringent controls of methadone use and restricts its dispensing to practitioners who are registered with DEA and in compliance with the Drug Abuse Prevention and Control Act.

The Drug Addiction Treatment Act of 2000 (DATA 2000) provides a waiver from the NATA requirements and permits qualified office-based physicians to prescribe and pharmacists to dispense schedule III, IV, or V narcotic drugs, or combinations of such drugs, approved by the FDA for the treatment of opioid addiction. In order to qualify for a waiver under DATA 2000, physicians must hold a current State medical license, a valid DEA registration number, and must meet one or more of the following conditions:

- The physician holds a subspecialty board certification in addiction psychiatry from the American Board of Medical Specialties.

- The physician holds an addiction certification from the American Society of Addiction Medicine.

- The physician holds a subspecialty board certification in addiction medicine from the American Osteopathic Association.

- The physician has completed not less than eight hours of training with respect to the treatment and management of opioid-addicted patients. This training can be provided through classroom situations, seminars at professional society meetings, electronic communications, or by other means. The training must be sponsored by one of five organizations authorized in the DATA 2000 legislation to sponsor such training, or by any other organization that the Secretary of the Department of Health and Human Services (the Secretary) determines to be appropriate.

- The physician has participated as an investigator in one or more clinical trials leading to the approval of a narcotic drug in Schedule III, IV, or V for maintenance or detoxification treatment, as demonstrated by a statement submitted to the Secretary by the sponsor of such approved drug.

- The physician has other training or experience, considered by the State medical licensing board (of the

State in which the physician will provide maintenance or detoxification treatment) to demonstrate the ability of the physician to treat and manage opioid-addicted patients.

- The physician has other training or experience that demonstrates the ability of the physician to treat and manage opioid-addicted patients.

In addition, physicians must attest that they have the capacity to refer addiction treatment patients for appropriate counseling and other non-pharmacological therapies, and that they will not have more than 30 patients on such addiction treatment at any one time. (Note: The patient limit applies to both physicians in solo practice and to entire group practices, and is not affected by the number of physician or group practice locations.)

Use of Buprenorphine Products

In Oct, 2002 The FDA approved the use of Subutex® (buprenorphine HCl) and Suboxone® (buprenorphine HCl + naloxone) sublingual tablets for the treatment of opioid dependence. Since both of these products contain buprenorphine HCl, a Schedule III drug, qualified office-based practitioners may prescribe it under the DATA 2000 regulations. It is recommended that Subutex® be given during the first few days of treatment, while Suboxone® be used during the maintenance phase of treatment.

Practitioner Requirements

With the exception of the waivers provided by the DATA 2000 regulations, all practitioners who intend to dispense or administer drugs in the treatment of opioid addiction are required to first obtain from the Secretary or by delegation, from the Administrator of the Substance Abuse and Mental Health Services Administration (SAMHSA), a certification that the practitioner is qualified under the Secretary's standards and will comply with such standards. Eligibility for certification depends upon the practitioner obtaining accreditation from an accreditation body that had been approved by SAMHSA. The regulations detail the procedures by which an entity can apply to become an approved accreditation body.

An exception to this registration requirement, known as the "three day rule", allows a practitioner who is not separately registered as a narcotic treatment program, to administer (but not prescribe) narcotic drugs to a patient for the purpose of relieving acute withdrawal symptoms while arranging for the patient's referral for treatment, under the following conditions:

- Not more than one day's medication may be administered or given to a patient at one time;
- This treatment may not be carried out for more than 72 hours and;
- This 72-hour period cannot be renewed or extended

The "three day rule" is intended to provide the practitioner with flexibility in emergency situations where he or she may be confronted with a patient undergoing acute withdrawal.

Practitioner Record Keeping Requirements

DEA record keeping requirements for office-based opioid therapy go beyond the Schedule III record keeping requirements. According to the DEA:

- Practitioners are required to keep records for controlled substances dispensed.
- Practitioners must keep records for controlled substances prescribed and dispensed to patients for maintenance or detoxification treatment, and
- Practitioners should keep separate records for these patients.

Standards for Federal Opioid Treatment Programs

The organizational structure and facilities of opioid treatment programs (OTPs) must be adequate to ensure quality patient care and to meet the requirements of all pertinent federal, state, and local laws and regulations. At a minimum, each OTP must formally designate a Program Sponsor and Medical Director. The Program Sponsor must agree, on behalf of the OTP, to adhere to all legal requirements dealing with the use of opioid agonist treatment medications in the treatment of opioid addiction.

The Medical Director of the OTP must assume responsibility for administering all medical services performed by the OTP. In addition, the Medical Director must be responsible for ensuring that the OTP is in compliance with all applicable federal, state, and local laws and regulations.

An OTP must maintain current quality assurance and quality control plans that include, among other things, annual reviews of program policies and procedures and on-going assessment of patient outcomes.

An OTP must maintain a current ``Diversion Control Plan'' (DCP) as part of its quality assurance program. The DCP must include specific measures to reduce the possibility of diversion of controlled substances from legitimate treatment use. It should also assign specific responsibility for carrying out the diversion control measures and functions described in the DCP to the medical and administrative staff of the OTP.

Each person engaged in the treatment of opioid addiction must have sufficient education, training, and experience, or any combination thereof, to enable that person to perform the assigned functions. All physicians, nurses, and other licensed professional care providers, including addiction counselors, must comply with the credentialing requirements of their respective professions.

An OTP must maintain current procedures designed to ensure that patients are admitted to maintenance treatment by qualified personnel who have determined, using accepted medical criteria such as those listed in the Diagnostic and Statistical Manual for Mental Disorders (DSM-IV), that the person is currently addicted to an opioid drug, and that the person became addicted at least one year before admission for treatment. In addition, a program physician must ensure that each patient has voluntarily chosen maintenance treatment and that all relevant facts concerning the use of the opioid drug are clearly and adequately explained to the patient. Each patient is also required to provide informed written consent for treatment.

A person under 18 years of age is required to have had two documented unsuccessful attempts at short-term detoxification or drug-free treatment within a **12**-month period to be eligible for maintenance treatment. No person under 18 years of age may be admitted to maintenance treatment unless a parent, legal guardian, or responsible adult designnated by the relevant state authority consents in writing to such treatment.

If clinically appropriate, the program physician may waive the requirement of a one year history of addiction for patients released from penal institutions (within 6 months after release), for pregnant patients (program physician must certify pregnancy), and for previously treated patients (up to 2 years after discharge).

Patients with two or more unsuccessful detoxification episodes within a **12**-month period must be assessed by the OTP physician for other forms of treatment. A program shall not admit a patient for more than two detoxification treatment episodes in one year.

Required Services for OTPs

OTPs must provide adequate medical, counseling, vocational, educational, and other assessment and treatment services. These services must be available at the primary facility, except where the program sponsor has entered into a formal, documented agreement with a private or public agency, organization, practitioner, or institution to provide these services to patients enrolled in the OTP. The program sponsor, in any event, must be able to document that these services are fully and reasonably available to patients.

OTPs must use only those opioid agonist treatment medications that are approved by the Food and Drug Administration for use in the treatment of opioid addiction. In addition, OTPs who are fully compliant with the protocol of an investigational use of a drug and other conditions set forth in the application may administer a drug that has been authorized by the Food and Drug Administration under an investigational new drug application for investigational use in the treatment of opioid addiction. Currently, the following narcotic agents are approved by the Food and Drug Administration for use in the treatment of opioid addiction:

- Methadone
- Levomethadyl acetate (LAAM, Orlaam)
- Buprenorphine HCl (Subutex, Suboxone)

OTPs must maintain current procedures that are adequate to ensure that the following dosage form and initial dosing requirements are met:

- Methadone or LAAM must be administered or dispensed only in oral form and must be formulated in such a way as to reduce their potential for parenteral abuse. Practitioners may not prescribe these agents for treatment of drug dependence.

- For each new patient enrolled in a program, the initial dose of methadone shall not exceed 30 milligrams and the total dose for the first day shall not exceed 40 milligrams, unless the program physician documents in the patient's record that 40 milligrams did not suppress opiate abstinence symptoms.

Dosing and administration decisions in the use of these drugs must be made by a program physician familiar with the most up-to-date product labeling. These procedures must ensure that any significant deviations from the approved labeling, including deviations with regard to dose, frequency, or the conditions of use described in the approved labeling, are specifically documented in the patient's record.

Prevention of Drug Diversion

To limit the potential for diversion of opioid agonist treatment medications to the illicit market, opioid agonist treatment medications dispensed to patients for unsupervised use shall be subject to the following requirements:

- Any patient in comprehensive maintenance treatment program may receive a single take-home dose for a day that the clinic is closed for business, including Sundays and state and federal holidays.

- Treatment program decisions for dispensing opioid treatment medications to patients for unsupervised use must be determined by the Medical Director. In determining which patients may be permitted unsupervised use, the Medical Director must consider the following take-home criteria in determining whether a patient is responsible in handling opioid drugs for unsupervised use.

  o Absence of recent abuse of drugs (opioid or nonnarcotic), including alcohol;
  o Regularity of clinic attendance;
  o Absence of serious behavioral problems at the clinic;

- o   Absence of known recent criminal activity, e.g., drug dealing;
- o   Stability of the patient's home environment and social relationships;
- o   Length of time in comprehensive maintenance treatment;
- o   Assurance that take-home medication can be safely stored within the patient's home; and
- o   Whether the rehabilitative benefit the patient derived from decreasing the frequency of clinic attendance outweighs the potential risks of diversion.

If it is determined that a patient is responsible in handling opioid drugs, the following restrictions apply:

- During the first 90 days of treatment, the take-home supply is limited to a single dose each week and the patient shall ingest all other doses under appropriate supervision.
- In the second 90 days of treatment, the take-home supply is two doses per week.
- In the third 90 days of treatment, the take-home supply is three doses per week.
- In the remaining months of the first year, a patient may be given a maximum 6-day supply of take-home medication.
- After one year of continuous treatment, a patient may be given a maximum 2-week supply of take-home medication.
- After two years of continuous treatment, a patient may be given a maximum one-month supply of take-home medication, but must make monthly visits.

No medications may be dispensed to patients in short-term detoxification treatment or interim maintenance treatment for unsupervised or take-home use.

OTPs must maintain current procedures adequate to identify the theft or diversion of take-home medications, including labeling containers with the OTP's name, address, and telephone number. Programs also must ensure that take-home supplies are packaged in a manner that is designed to reduce the risk of accidental ingestion, including the use of child-resistant containers.

Section I

Nonprescription Drugs

General Labeling Requirements

Over-the-counter (OTC) or nonprescription status is granted to drugs and drug products that have been shown to be safe for use without a physician's supervision, are for conditions suitable for self-diagnosis, and have adequate written directions for self-use. Of major importance with OTC products is appropriate labeling. This refers to label terminology that is easily understood by the general public.

Federal law requires manufacturers to use a "seven-point" label on nonprescription products. Included on the label must be:

- name of the product
- name and address of the manufacturer, packer, or distributor
- net contents of the package

- established name of all active ingredients and certain inactive ingredients
- name of any habit-forming drug present
- cautions and warnings needed to protect the consumer
- adequate directions for use

If any of the above information is missing, the nonprescription product is considered misbranded.

Other required information on nonprescription product labeling may include:

- a statement of the intended use of the drug (e.g. "for motion sickness").
- dosage range appropriate for different ages
- how often the OTC may be safely taken
- route or method of administration
- other factors that may affect the efficacy of the drug (example: "take before meals" or "take one hour before bedtime")

In March 1999 the FDA published new OTC regulations. The stated objective of the new legislation was to allow consumers to better understand OTC information. The law provides that labels of nonprescription drug products must present "Drug Facts" in a standard order (similar to the "Nutrition Facts" on food products). The order of presentation recommended is:

- active ingredients
- purpose
- uses

- warnings
- directions
- other information
- inactive ingredients

Figure I-1 is an example of this new "Drug Facts" section.

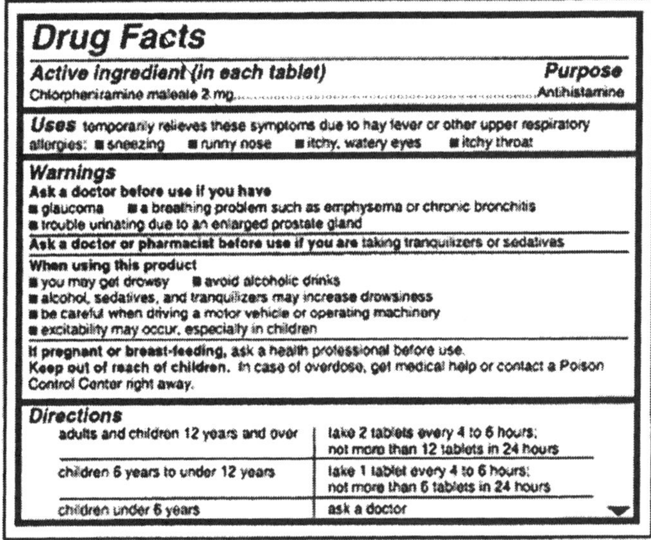

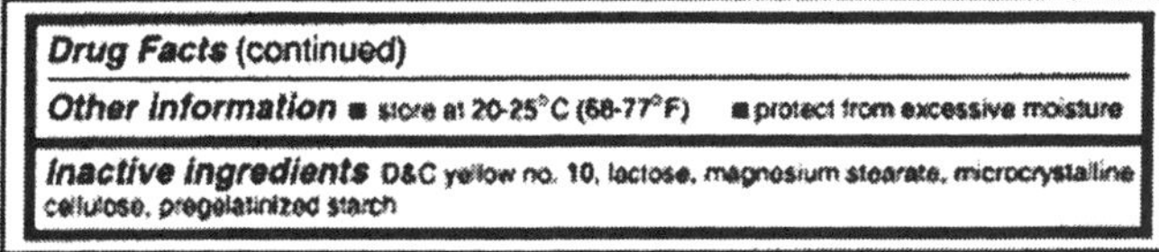

Figure I-1. Example of new Drug Facts section of Nonprescription product labeling.

The legislation also provides that the warnings section of nonprescription labels include the statement "Ask your doctor or pharmacist about food or drug interactions." In addition, the simplified standard language on OTC labels includes the term "uses", not "indications". Use of the terms "precautions" and "contraindications" are also eliminated.

OTC Labeling for Pregnancy and Nursing Mothers

Federal regulations mandate labeling for non-prescription drug products intended for systemic use. The general warning states: "As with any drug, if you are pregnant or nursing a baby, seek the advice of a health professional before using this product". Exceptions to this labeling will include those drugs intended to benefit the fetus or nursing infant and those products intended exclusively for pediatric use.

Some OTC drugs such as oral or rectal products containing aspirin must have the warning: "It is especially important not to use this product during the last three months of pregnancy unless specifically directed to do so by a doctor".

OTC Labeling of Sodium Content

Federal regulations require that the labeling for OTC products intended for oral administration must indicate the sodium content per dosage unit (i.e., per teaspoonful, tablespoonful, etc.), if the amount present exceeds 5 mg per single dose. This total refers to all sources of sodium whether present in active or inactive ingredients.

If the amount of sodium per dosage unit is greater than 140 mg, a warning on the label must state: "Do not use this product if you are on a sodium restricted diet unless recommended by a doctor".

Acceptable terminology indicating sodium levels is specified in Figure I-2.

Figure I-2. Meaning of OTC Sodium Level Designations

Designation	Meaning
Sodium Free	Contains less than 0.5 mg of sodium per dosage unit
Very Low Sodium	Contains 35 mg or less of sodium per dosage unit
Low Sodium	Contains 140 mg or less of sodium per dosage unit

NOTE: All of the above quantities refer to the content of sodium, NOT sodium chloride.

OTC Labeling for Other Electrolytes

In 2004, the FDA issued rules for labeling other electrolytes present in OTC products. The label must indicate the presence of each of the following minerals if the level of the mineral in each dose is equal to or exceeds the threshold amount indicated:

Mineral	**Threshold Amount**
Calcium	0.2 mg
Magnesium	0.8 mg
Potassium	0.5 mg

In addition, label warnings intended for individuals on electrolyte-restricted diets are required if the maximum daily intake of a mineral will exceed the threshold amounts indicated below.

Mineral	**Threshold Amount**
Sodium	140 mg
Calcium	3.5 g
Magnesium	600 mg
Potassium	975 mg

Tamper-resistant Packaging

After several instances of deliberate addition of poisons to commercial nonprescription drug packages on store shelves, the Tamper-resistant Packaging Act was passed. The intent of this regulation is to prevent the intentional contamination of over-the-counter products.

Some exemptions from the requirement include:

- Aerosol products
- Nonprescription products not accessible to the general public (such as those in hospitals and other institutions)
- Lozenges, and drugs in first aid kits

In November 1998, the Act was clarified by using the term "Tamper-evident Packaging". It is intended to heighten consumer awareness of potential tampering, without implying that a particular package is difficult to open or that it is "tamper-proof".

This legislation also requires that two-piece hard gelatin capsules must be sealed using a tamper-evident technology and that the packages containing the capsules have at least one tamper-evident feature.

Prescription to OTC Reclassification

Requests for the reclassification of a prescription-only drug to OTC status are accomplished by one of the following four mechanisms:

- If the drug is now a prescription drug, a full NDA (New Drug Application) requesting OTC status may be submitted to the FDA for its evaluation.

- The FDA may grant an exemption if it deems that prescription-only status is unnecessary for the protection of the public health.

- A supplement to the NDA may be filed. The FDA will then review the relative safety of the drug based upon previous marketing experience and lack of a history of adverse effects.

- The Nonprescription Drug Advisory Committee may recommend that a particular ingredient be converted to nonprescription status.

The Nonprescription Drug Advisory Committees were originally established to evaluate the numerous nonprescription products and individual ingredients currently on the market. The committees or panels, subdivided by therapeutic categories, submitted their conclusions to the FDA. As a result of their deliberations, OTC ingredients were classified into one of three categories.

- **Category I**   Generally recognized as safe and effective (GRASE) for the claimed therapeutic indication

- **Category II**   Not generally recognized as safe and effective or having unacceptable indications

- **Category III**   Insufficient data available to permit final classification

Based upon data submitted or following the failure of companies to submit data, the status of specific OTC ingredients may be changed from one category to another. For example, in 2002, the FDA banned the use of aloe and cascara sagrada as laxative ingredients in over-the-counter drug products. These two groups of ingredients are deemed as not being GRASE (generally recognized as safe and effective). This effectively placed these ingredients into Category II. Laxative products containing any form of aloe or cascara sagrada are now considered to be misbranded.

> # Note
> Questions on either the NAPLEX® or the MPJE® may be designed to determine if the candidate is familiar with the status of a specific drug product. Drugs or drug products that were switched from Rx-only to nonprescription status within the past few years may be included. However, the exam will likely avoid including drug products whose status may change in the near future or those that are being presently evaluated for a change. It is unlikely that questions that ask for concentrations or strengths of prescription versus nonprescription products will be asked on the MPJE®.

Nonprescription Sale of Ipecac Syrup

While Ipecac Syrup contains the federal legend requiring dispensing only by prescription, there is one notable exception. A 30 mL container of Ipecac Syrup may be sold as a nonprescription item. The intent of this exemption is to provide every household with an emetic for the immediate treatment of accidental poisoning.

To qualify for nonprescription sale

- Only 30mL containers of Ipecac Syrup may be sold.

- The bottle label must state in red letters: "For emergency use to cause vomiting in poisoning. Before using, call a physician, the Poison Control Center, or a hospital emergency room immediately for advice."

- The label should contain the warning: "Keep out of reach of children. Do not use in unconscious persons." "Do not use when strychnine, corrosives such as alkalies and strong acids, or petroleum distillates such as kerosene, gasoline, fuel, oil, paint thinner, or cleaning fluid have been ingested".

- The usual dosage of Ipecac Syrup in persons over one year of age is one tablespoonful (15mL).

Sample Questions

1. The maximum volume of Ipecac Syrup that may be sold without a prescription is:
   (A) 15 mL   (B) 30 mL   (C) 60 mL
   (D) 120 mL   (E) > 120 mL

2. Under which of the following circumstances may Ipecac Syrup be sold without a prescription?

   I.   For future use during accidental poisoning
   II. Only if the household does not have small children
   III. If the purchaser signs a pharmacy logbook
   (A) I only   (B) III only   (C) I & II only
   (D) II & III only   (E) I, II, & III

3. The label of a bottle of Ipecac Syrup sold OTC for accidental poisoning must:
   I.   state that the appropriate dose is the entire bottle followed by a full glass of water.
   II. provide the telephone number of a poison control center.
   III. must have its warnings printed in red ink.

   (A) I only   (B) III only   (C) I & II only
   (D) II & III only   (E) I, II, & III

Answers: (1) B   (2) A   (3) B

Nonprescription Sale of Quinine

In 1998, the FDA classified nonprescription quinine products to be unsafe for the treatment and/or prevention of malaria. Previously the use of nonprescription quinine products for nocturnal leg cramps was discontinued because there was a lack of substantial evidence of its effectiveness as well as concerns about potential toxicity.

Section J

Dietary and Nutritional Products

Dietary Supplement Health Education Act (DSHEA)

This act exempts health foods, food supplements, and herbal products from the strict controls imposed by the FDA on prescription drugs and OTC drug products. Products included under DSHEA are vitamins, minerals, herbals, amino acids and related supplements. Provisions of this act include the following:

- Products may be marketed without their efficacy proven. This means that the FTC or FDA would have to challenge products after they have been introduced onto the market if there is evidence that they are ineffective for the advertised or labeled use.

- Products currently on the market do not have to be proven safe. It is the responsibility of the FDA to prove that a product is unsafe before it can be challenged. However, the manufacturer must provide "reasonable" assurances that no ingredient in the product presents a significant or unreasonable risk of illness or injury.

- Product manufacturing processes do not have to meet FDA's GMPs. The FDA good manufacturing practices are very detailed and strict. To manufacture drug products, every pharmaceutical manufacturer must submit specific details of their production facilities and describe how every product is processed. This is not required for dietary supplements, herbals, etc. However, this does not mean that these products can be made under unsanitary conditions. At the present time, dietary supplement and herbal manufacturers are developing GMP guidelines for these products.

Manufacturers are permitted to make structure/function claims on labels if the statements do not indicate that the product will diagnose, cure, treat, or prevent a disease. Some claims related to the product's ability to affect body structure or function are permitted if they are truthful and not misleading. For example, a claim that Saw Palmetto will "improve urinary flow" or that it is "for the prostate" is acceptable. A statement such as "will cure an enlarged prostate" is not acceptable. While any product claims must be substantiated by the manufacturer, they do NOT have to be reviewed or approved by the FDA. The manufacturer must state this fact (i.e. that the FDA has not reviewed product claims) on the label.

Official Status of Herbals

The USP/NF has developed monographs for some botanicals that appear to have therapeutic activity. To be admitted into the USP, the herb must have an FDA approved use or a USP DI Panel recognized use. At the present time, the active herbs have not been admitted to the USP, but have been admitted to the NF when there are no significant safety concerns. The monographs describe the portions of plant used, its botanical characteristics, and appropriate assay procedures for ingredients. The monographs do not describe the therapeutic uses of the herb. Monographs are currently available for chamomile, cranberry liquid preparation, feverfew, garlic, ginger, ginkgo, milk thistle, St John's wort, saw palmetto, and valerian.

Note

Since there is an ongoing dialogue between the FDA and manufacturers of the above products as to the interpretation of allowable claims, it is unlikely any specific questions about these products will appear on the MPJE®.

Ban on Sales of Ephedra and Ephedrine Alkaloids

For centuries ephedra has been used for several indications including asthma. However, in 2004 the FDA banned the sales of all dietary supplements containing this drug, citing that its use posed an unreasonable risk of illness or injury to consumers. Based upon the DSHEA (Dietary Supplement Health and Education Act), the FDA claimed that dietary supplements containing ephedra or its alkaloids are adulterated since they present an unreasonable risk of illness or injury based upon their recommended use.

The ban does not apply to prescription or non-prescription drug products or to conventional foods such as herbal teas. It also does not apply to products that are prepared or used for "Traditional Chinese Medicine" since this practice uses ephedra for temporary respiratory conditions, not for chronic, long-term use for weight loss. In addition, the product labels must not have any indication that the product is a dietary supplement.

Sample Questions

Answer the following questions using the key of:
(A) I only   (B) III only   (C) I & II only
(D) II & III only   (E) I, II, & III

1.   Which of the following statements is (are) true?
   I.   None of the herbals used in the US are recognized in the USP/NF.
   II.   Commercial herbals may be categorized as nonprescription drugs.
   III. Commercial herbals are categorized as dietary supplements.

2.   A pharmacist may sell herbals provided that:
   I.   The patient is properly counseled with respect to their use.
   II.   The consumer is cautioned to use the product for not more than two weeks.
   III.   There are adequate directions on the package for patient use.

3.   Upon formal request, to whom must the manufacturer of an herbal product submit data supporting the claims for the product?
I.   FDA or FTC
II.   pharmacists
III.   consumers

Answers: (1) B   (2) B   (3) A

Homeopathic Drug Products

The Federal Food, Drug and Cosmetic Act of 1938 recognized the Homeopathic Pharmacopoeia of the United States (HPUS) as an official compendium. Drug products that use an official name designation found in the HPUS must meet all of its compendial standards. Otherwise the drug product is misbranded or adulterated.

The basic elements of homeopathic medicine include individualized dosing of patients by homeopathic physicians, based upon a patient's symptoms. The dose of drug administered is usually extremely low; often dilutions of 1:1,000 or 1:1,000,000 are used with frequent drug administration. These drug products must meet the usual drug labeling requirements including ingredient names, amounts, and directions for use. While many of the drugs were originally labeled by their Latin name, it is now required that their English name be provided. Some of the drugs found in homeopathic formulas are also official in the USP/NF. In these situations, the drug must meet the stricter standards found in the USP/NF. If the drug product is intended for nonprescription use, its label must include appropriate warning statements, if needed.

While homeopathic drugs must be manufactured under GMP standards, they do not have to have an expiration date on their package.

Section K

Cosmetics

The legal distinction between cosmetics and drugs is somewhat muddled. For example, some cosmetics, such as fluoridated toothpaste, medicated mouthwash, or anti-dandruff shampoos are borderline between being classified as cosmetics versus nonprescription products. The overriding factor in determining a product's status may not be its ingredients, but what claims are made for the product, especially on the label. Unlike drugs, cosmetics do not require premarketing approval from the FDA.

While cosmetic manufacturers do not have to meet the rigorous requirements of the FDA's Good Manufacturing Practice (GMP) program, they are still obligated to manufacture these products under sanitary conditions. Otherwise, the products may be considered to be adulterated. While the Federal Food, Drug, and Cosmetic Act of 1938 does not specifically state that cosmetics have to be tested for safety, any cosmetic that poses a safety problem to the general public will be considered as being misbranded. If an unapproved color additive is used in the formulation, the product will be classified as being adulterated.

Regulation of advertising and labeling of cosmetics basically falls under the jurisdiction of the Federal Trade Commission (FTC). The labels of cosmetic products must contain the names of ingredients listed in descending order of predominance (that is why water may be listed as the first ingredient, while the "active ingredient" is listed further down in the ingredient list). Ingredients present in quantities of one percent or less may be listed at the bottom, in random order. Perfumes and flavoring oils may simply be listed by name. Coloring agents must be those accepted for cosmetic use. A minor exception to the above ingredient listing requirement are cosmetics used in professional settings such as by professional hairdressers (i.e. cosmetics not intended for retail sales).

The ingredient names listed on labels must be the generic names listed in the USP/NF. If an ingredient is not of USP/NF quality or not listed in these two official books, other relevant sources such as the *CTFA Cosmetic Ingredient Dictionary* may be used. This book has been compiled by the Cosmetic, Toiletry, and Fragrance Association (CTFA) and contains many ingredients commonly used in cosmetics (e.g. surfactants).

Many cosmetic products, especially those intended for use in body cavities (e.g. mouthwashes and vaginal products) must be packaged in tamper-resistant packaging.

Sample Questions

1. Which one of the following organizations is responsible for establishing names for ingredients used in cosmetic formulations?
   (A) ASHP   (B) APhA   (C) CTFA
   (D) HCFA   (E) RDA

2. A client in a pharmacy complains about her hypersensitivity to many ingredients found in cosmetic lotions When reading the label of a sunscreen lotion, which one of the following ingredients is not required to be listed by the manufacturer?
   (A)   antimicrobial preservative
   (B)   coloring agent
   (C)   sunscreening agent
   (D)   perfuming oil
   (E)   water

3. The general guideline for listing ingredients on a cosmetic product label consists of listing the additives
   (A)   and active ingredients intermixed but in the alphabetical sequence.
   (B)   and active ingredients intermixed but ranked by decreasing concentrations.
   (C)   and active ingredients intermixed but ranked by increasing concentrations.
   (D)   listed separately from the active ingredients.
   (E)   listed separately by decreasing concentrations.

4. A cosmetic hand lotion consists of an oil-in-water emulsion. The first ingredient listed on its label is most likely to be the:
   (A) oil that is present   (B) perfume
   (C) coloring agent   (D) surfactant
   (E) water

Answers: (1) C   (2) D   (3) B   (4) E

Section L

Miscellaneous Laws and Regulations

Alcohol Regulations

The Bureau of Alcohol, Tobacco and Firearms controls the sale of alcohol. Pharmacies may purchase 95% ethanol (190 proof grain alcohol) for routine compounding by using Form ATF-11. If a pharmacy is selling alcohol in the form of a beverage, it must obtain a retail liquor dealer's stamp. Institutions that have a need for greater volumes of alcohol may choose to purchase tax-free alcohol, since it is much lower in cost (tax on regular alcohol purchases is very high). Such pharmacies must purchase alcohol by using Form ATF-1447.

The following are federal statutes that relate to the use of tax-free alcohol:

- Its use is limited to medicinal or scientific use, or in patient treatment.

- The alcohol may not be sold or loaned to other pharmacies or physician's offices.

- The alcohol, either by itself or as a component of other products, may not be sold to outpatients. An exception to this requirement permits nonprofit clinics to dispense medicines made with tax-free alcohol provided the client is not charged for the medication.

- A running, accurate inventory must be kept for all alcohol in stock.

- Containers of alcohol, usually supplied in 10 or 55 gallon drums, must be stored in a securely locked, fire-resistant storeroom.

How may a prescriber's order for an alcohol-containing beverage (e.g. brandy at bedtime) for an institutionalized client be handled? Either

- the institution may buy the alcohol-containing beverage, furnish it to the client, and then bill the patient.

- the hospital pharmacy may give the patient's relatives permission to bring in alcohol for the patient.

Another available form of tax-exempt alcohol is Specially Denatured Alcohol (SDA). SDAs refers to specific formulas of grain (ethyl) alcohol that have been rendered unsuitable for use as a beverage by the addition of denaturants such as sucrose octaacetate, brucine, or butyl alcohol. There are a large number of formulas for SDAs, usually designated as SDA 40A, SDA 23H, etc. SDAs are often used for pharmaceutical processing and in commercial products such as mouthwashes.

Americans with Disabilities Act (ADA)

The Federal Rehabilitation Act of 1973 prevents an employer from discriminating against a handicapped person who is otherwise qualified to perform the functions of a job. The Act applies only to those companies receiving federal assistance. The employee's handicap could be either mental or physical. The Americans with Disabilities Act (ADA) was passed in 1990 with an effective date of 1992. This act expands the original Rehabilitation Act by greatly increasing the number of individuals covered and by covering companies even if they are not receiving federal financial assistance. Any company employing 15 or more people is covered. In both acts, the term "disabled" is used since it has less of a negative connotation than the term "handicapped".

These acts provide civil rights protection to individuals with disabilities similar to those provided to individuals on the basis of race, color, sex, national origin, age, and religion. Among those covered under the ADA are individuals with epilepsy, paralysis, HIV infections, AIDS, mental retardation, and alcoholics. Those NOT protected are individuals who illegally use drugs. A key concept of both acts is that employers must make a "reasonable effort" to accommodate a disabled employee.

The following are additional elements of these laws:

- The employer must make reasonable accommodations for disabled individuals whether those individuals are employees or members of the general public. For the general public, "reasonable accommodations" include providing ramps leading into a building, providing elevator service to all floors of a building, and constructing restroom facilities that are accessible to disabled individuals.

- For an employee, "reasonable accommodations" might include a reduced-height workbench.

- An employer may not ask about disabilities during an employment interview, but may ask if the prospective employee has the ability to perform the work.

Note

A court has ruled that pharmacists who are HIV positive may not be discriminated against by either refusing them employment or by refusing to assign them to the usual daily functions of a pharmacist. This concept could be extended to pregnant female pharmacists who may wish to prepare chemotherapy drug admixtures. Obviously if they prefer NOT to work with potential mutagenic agents, their wishes should be honored.

- An employer may not require a prospective employee to undergo a medical examination before offering a position. However, the employer may require a medical examination as a condition of employment if this is a requirement for all new employees.

Note

Tests for illegal use of drugs are not considered to be medical examinations and may be required by an employer

Sample Questions

1. The requirements of the ADA must be followed if what minimum number of employees is employed in a pharmacy?
   (A) 2 (B) 10 (C) 15 (D) 50 (E) 100

2. Which of the following conditions may preclude a pharmacist from working in a hospital pharmacy?
   I.   alcoholism
   II. HIV infection
   III. cocaine addiction
   (A) I only   (B) III only   (C) I & II only
   (D) II & III only   (E) I, II, & III

3. An institutional pharmacy employer may NOT prevent pharmacists with which of the following conditions from working in a parenteral admixture room?
   I.   chronic alcoholism
   II. HIV infection
   III. epilepsy
   (A) I only   (B) III only   (C) I & II only
   (D) II & III only   (E) I, II, & III

4. The ADA protects an employee if an employer attempts to enforce:
   I.   random locker-room searches for illegal drugs
   II. IQ tests
   III. weight reduction programs
   (A) I only   (B) III only   (C) I & II only
   (D) II & III only   (E) I, II, & III

Answers: (1) C   (2) B   (3) E   (4) D

E-mail use in Pharmacy Practice

A federal law passed in December, 2003 affects all unsolicited commercial e-mailing. The law's intent is to reduce unsolicited e-mailing (spam) from all sources. All companies that issue e-mail messages must identify themselves within the message and provide physical address contact information. In addition, the subject line of the e-mail must be truthful and not deceptive.

Other requirements of this law specify that each commercial e-mail message must:

- identify itself as an advertisement or solicitation.
- originate from a legitimate e-mail address to which a recipient may reply.
- be sent from a legitimate domain name and have correct header information that allows tracing to its origin.
- have a mechanism by which a recipient may choose not to receive future messages.

Drug-free Workplace

According to the Federal Anti-Drug Abuse Act of 1988

- The unlawful possession of controlled substances by employees is prohibited in the workplace.

- If an employee is convicted of criminal possession of drugs, he/she must inform the employer of the conviction within five days.

*   Employers may take appropriate action.

Unfair Competition

It is unlikely that questions concerning the economic aspects of pharmacy will be asked on the MPJE®. However, one should be aware of two major laws in this area.

Sherman Antitrust Act

The Sherman Antitrust Act prevents restraint of trade or the establishment of monopolies. Originally, the Sherman Antitrust Act was intended to curtail the large monopolies that operated in the early 1900's. The concept of the Act is to prevent restraint of trade and/or the establishment of monopolies. Companies or groups may not have agreements, either formal or informal, among themselves, which would unreasonably restrain trade. For example, three independent pharmacies in a given area may not agree to a common drug mark-up of 40% or a professional fee of $15.00. These actions would probably be classified as price fixing. Other examples could be the distribution of suggested retail prices for certain prescription drugs by a pharmaceutical organization or the boycott by a group of pharmacies of a third party payer because of its low reimbursement rate. In addition, a group of pharmacies may not agree as a group to reject a third-party prescription plan, nor can they collectively bargain for better reimbursement rates. However, a chain consisting of several pharmacies may do so.

Robinson-Patman Act

The intent of the Robinson-Patman Act is to prevent the hindering of competition. A seller is not allowed to practice price discrimination when dealing with similar purchasers. For example, the wholesale price for 100 x 1,000 tablet bottles may not favor one pharmacy over another. Likewise, this issue arises when individual states allow hospitals to dispense prescriptions to walk-in clients if the hospital has a community pharmacy permit. In this case, however, the price of the prescription may not be based upon the special, reduced price that the hospital receives from the pharmaceutical manufacturer. Nor can the hospital sell drugs or medical devices to affiliated groups such as a home health care business at the special, reduced price.

Hospitals and similar institutions do have the right to extend their special prices to employees, inpatients, emergency room patients, etc. This is known as "own use". Institutions are not permitted to provide prescription refills for former patients unless the take-home drugs are intended as continued care or are supplementing treatment administered in the hospital (e.g. continuing a treatment with parenteral antibiotics).

While physicians on the hospital staff may be supplied with drugs for personal use, drugs may not be sold to physicians for use in their private practice, especially if the drugs are being sold to patients.

Section M

Sample Questions

1.   Which of the following are Schedule I controlled sub-
       stances?
       I.   mescaline
       II.   peyote
       III. heroin
       (A) I only   (B) III only   (C) I & II only
       (D) II & III only   (E) I, II, & III

2.   Which of the products listed below would be considered
       to be Schedule III controlled substances?
       I.   A product that contains 90 mg of codeine per
             dose
       II.   A product that contains 15 mg of hydrocodone
             per dose
       III. A product that contains 2.5 mg of diphenoxylate and
             25 mcg of atropine sulfate per dose
       (A) I only   (B) III only   (C) I & II only
       (D) II & III only   (E) I, II, & III

3.   Primary responsibility for oversight of nonprescription
       drug advertising rests with the
       (A) FDA   (B) FTC   (C) HCFA
       (D) DEA   (E) USP/NF

4.   Partial filling of a schedule IV controlled substance
       prescription is permissible, provided that
       I.   each partial filling is recorded.
       II.   the total quantity dispensed in all partial fillings
             does not exceed the total quantity prescribed.
       III. the total price charged for the partial fillings
             does not exceed the total price the patient
             would have paid with a complete filling of the
             prescription.
       (A) I only   (B) III only   (C) I & II only
       (D) II & III only   (E) I, II, & III

5.   When a pharmacist conducts a controlled substance
       inventory, which of the following must be included?
       I.   Drugs stored in a warehouse for the registrant
             at a different location.
       II.   Drugs ordered by a customer but not yet paid
             for.
       III. All controlled substances dispensed over the
             past 30 days.
       (A) I only   (B) III only   (C) I & II only
       (D) II & III only   (E) I, II, & III

6.   Which of the following are Schedule IV controlled
       substances?
       I.   mazindol
       II.   fenfluramine
       III. buprenorphine
       (A) I only   (B) III only   (C) I & II only
       (D) II & III only   (E) I, II, & III

7.   A "Listed Chemical" is defined by the Controlled
       Substances Act as any chemical that is
       (A)   a controlled substance
       (B)   listed in the USP/NF
       (C)   listed in the USP DI
       (D)   used in manufacturing a controlled substance
       (E)   listed in the Orange Book

8. The pharmacist counsels a customer concerning the purchase of a body lotion which does not contain the coloring agent, tartrazine, to which she is allergic. While examining product labels with the client, the pharmacist should explain that:
   I. rather than list each individual coloring agent, the manufacturer may simply list "yellow dye".
   II. the ingredients, including tartrazine, will be listed alphabetically.
   III. the concentration of tartrazine present may not be listed.
   (A) I only   (B) III only   (C) I & II only
   (D) II & III only   (E) I, II, & III

9. Which of the following conditions must exist for the inspection of a pharmacy by an authorized inspector?
   I. Inspection must be conducted during the regular business hours of the pharmacy
   II. The owner of the pharmacy or the designated supervising pharmacist must be present
   III. The inspector must have a search warrant
   (A) I only   (B) III only   (C) I & II only
   (D) II & III only   (E) I, II, & III

10. A pharmacist telephones a patient's home concerning the availability of a prescription refill. With which of the following parties may the message be left?
    I. patient's wife
    II. patient's mother
    III. patient's brother-in-law
    (A) I only   (B) III only   (C) I & II only
    (D) II & III only   (E) I, II, & III

11. The selling of drug samples in pharmacies is prohibited by which one of the following Federal acts?
    (A) DSHEA
    (B) Durham Humphrey
    (C) Prescription Drug Marketing Act
    (D) Sherman Act
    (E) Drug Price Competition Act

12. Which of the following statements concerning bar coding of prescription drug labels is(are) accurate?
    I. The drug name and strength must be included in the bar code.
    II. The products expiration date may be included in the bar code.
    III. Labels of vaccine products must be bar coded.
    (A) I only   (B) III only   (C) I & II only
    (D) II & III only   (E) I, II, & III

13. According to FDA guidelines, which of the following activities are NOT acceptable for an individual receiving mailed prescription drugs from a Canadian pharmacy?
    I. Splitting the drug supply with his neighbor who also has a prescription for the same product.
    II. Receiving a six months supply of the drug
    III. Having the drug mailed directly to his home rather than to his physician
    (A) I only   (B) III only   (C) I & II only
    (D) II & III only   (E) I, II, & III

14. Which of the following is true of dispensing controlled substance-containing products without a prescription?
    I. Not more than 120 mL or 24 dosage units of Robitussin A-C cough medicine may be dispensed in any given 48-hour period.
    II. Not more than 240mL or 48 dosage units of Camphorated Opium Tincture (Paregoric) may be dispensed in any given 48-hour period.
    III. The purchaser must be at least 21 years of age
    (A) I only   (B) III only   (C) I & II only
    (D) II & III only   (E) I, II, & III

15. Schedule III, IV, and V controlled substance prescriptions may be issued to a community pharmacy pursuant to
    I.   a fax of a written, signed prescription transmitted by the prescriber to the pharmacy
    II. an oral prescription called in by a prescriber
    III. a written prescription signed by the prescriber
    (A) I only   (B) III only   (C) I & II only
    (D) II & III only   (E) I, II, & III

16. The requirement for over-the-counter drugs to have "adequate directions for use"
    (A)   means that the directions will be clear to a layperson for safe use of the product.
    (B)   applies only to products intended for oral consumption
    (C)   applies only to products for pediatric use
    (D)   includes the listing of potential side effects and toxicity
    (E)   includes the presence of bilingual directions

17. The label of a parenteral product is not required to list the presence of a(an):
    (A)   antimicrobial preservative
    (B)   buffer system
    (C)   inert gas
    (D)   antioxidant
    (E)   chelating agent

18. A pharmaceutical manufacturer has withdrawn a drug from the market since it was deemed by the FDA to be ineffective. Under which one of the following conditions may a pharmacy volunteer to compound capsules of the drug for patients?

(A)   if only 14 day supplies of the capsules are dispensed

(B)   if a physician writes the prescription specifying "medically necessary"

(C)   if the capsule strength is one-half or less than the original commercial capsule

(D)   only specific physicians write for the prescriptions

(E)   if the pharmacy is willing to be cited for violations of FDA guidelines for compounding

19.   A pharmacy has been compounding a psoriasis cream in 30 gram jars based upon prescriptions written by physicians in a dermatology clinic. Under which of the following circumstances could the pharmacy also dispense the jars?

I.   For patients of other prescribers based upon written prescriptions

II.   To the original dermatology clinic for dispensing by the dermatologists

III.   To other pharmacies provided they provide a written purchase order

(A) I only   (B) III only   (C) I & II only
(D) II & III only   (E) I, II, & III

20.   The SMART program is intended to assure appropriate and safe dispensing of which one of the following drugs?

(A) aspirin   (B) isotretinoin   (C) nevirapine
(D) sildenafil   (E) thalidomide

21.   Which of the following prescriptions for Accutane must bear the yellow sticker?

I.   Rx for an unmarried 16 year-old female
II.   Rx for a 60 year-old female
III.   Rx for a 30 year-old male

(A) I only   (B) III only   (C) I & II only
(D) II & III only   (E) I, II, & III

22. Labels of OTC products that are for systemic absorption
    must include a warning specifically intended to protect:
    I.   pregnant women
    II. nursing women
    III. geriatric women
    (A) I only   (B) III only   (C) I & II only
    (D) II & III only   (E) I, II, & III

23. Which of the following are NOT controlled substances?
    I.   ergotamine tartrate
    II. papaverine
    III. levorphanol
    (A) I only   (B) III only   (C) I & II only
    (D) II & III only   (E) I, II, & III

24. Pharmacists are required to periodically inventory
    supplies of which of the following drug products?
    I.   phenobarbital elixir
    II. Entex Liquid
    III. Sudafed Plus Liquid
    (A) I only   (B) III only   (C) I & II only
    (D) II & III only   (E) I, II, & III

25. In 2002, the FDA ruled that the nonprescription drug
    ingredient, cascara sagrada belongs in the OTC
    Category II. Products containing this ingredient
    will be considered by the FDA to be:
    (A) adulterated   (B) expired   (C) misbranded
    (D) potentially toxic   (E) safe and effective

26. Refusal of a patient to provide medical information for a
    patient prescription profile means that the pharmacist:
    I.   can fill the prescription at his/her discretion.
    II. must call the patient's physician to confirm the
         patient's medical condition
    III. must tell the patient that the prescription may not be
         filled without the requested information.
    (A) I only   (B) III only   (C) I & II only
    (D) II & III only   (E) I, II, & III

27.   While presenting a talk on drug abuse, a pharmacist is asked for information concerning the "date-rape drug". Her response may include which of following?
I.   The drug is a Schedule II substance.
II.   The generic name for the drug is gamma-hydroxybutyric acid
III.   The therapeutic classification of the drug is as a behavioral depressant and hypnotic.
(A) I only   (B) III only   (C) I & II only
(D) II & III only   (E) I, II, & III

28.   Which one of the following must be present on the labels of nonprescription drug products intended for oral use?
(A)   sodium content of active ingredients
(B)   total sodium content of both active and inactive ingredients
(C)   sodium chloride content of active ingredients
(D)   total sodium chloride content of both active and inactive ingredients
(E)   no requirements have been established

29.   Which of the following are included in the FDA's 2004 ban on sales of products containing ephedra?
I.   Amobarbital
II.   Pentobarbital
III.   Phenobarbital
(A) I only   (B) III only   (C) I & II only
(D) II & III only   (E) I, II, & III

30.   The organization responsible for overseeing the selection of a nonproprietary name for a new drug is the:
(A) FDA   (B) FTC   (C) USAN
(D) USP/NF   (E) APhA

31. Which of the following are examples of Schedule I
    substances?
    I.   Lysergic acid diethylamide
    II. Mescaline
    III. Peyote
    (A) I only   (B) III only   (C) I & II only
    (D) II & III only   (E) I, II, & III

32. A new drug product is given the name "felorazepam". It
    is likely to be classified as
    (A) Schedule II   (B) Schedule III   (C) Schedule IV
    (D) ScheduleV   (E) Noncontrolled

33. Which of the following barbiturates is classified in
    controlled substance category IV?
    I.   Amobarbital
    II. Pentobarbital
    III. Phenobarbital
    (A) I only   (B) III only   (C) I & II only
    (D) II & III only   (E) I, II, & III

34. A new cough syrup contains 15 mg of codeine phosphate
    and 100 mg of guaifenesin in each 10 mL dose. A 4 fluid
    ounce container of this product would likely be classified
    as
    (A) Schedule II   (B) Schedule III   (C) Schedule IV
    (D) ScheduleV   (E) Noncontrolled

35. How may a physician obtain cocaine HCl powder for
    use as a local anesthetic in his office?
    I.   He may write a prescription for the drug and
         write "for office use" on its face.
    II. He may write an order for the drug in an
         institutional setting and label it "for office use"
    III. He may order it directly from a supplier using
         DEA Form 222.
    (A) I only   (B) III only   (C) I & II only
    (D) II & III only   (E) I, II, & III

36.   A pharmacist may issue a Power of Attorney to an individual in order to permit the individual to
I.   fill controlled substance prescriptions.
II.   conduct a narcotic treatment facility.
III.   complete DEA Form 222 orders.
(A) I only   (B) III only   (C) I & II only
(D) II & III only   (E) I, II, & III

37.   A pharmacist who fills an oral morphine sulfate prescription in an emergency does not receive a "cover" prescription from the prescriber. The pharmacist must
I.   notify the regional DEA office.
II.   notify the state board of medicine.
III.   call the patient and request that he/she obtain a written prescription to cover the oral order.
(A) I only   (B) III only   (C) I & II only
(D) II & III only   (E) I, II, & III

38.   A physician wishes to prescribe a schedule II controlled substance for a patient residing in a hospice. How may the prescription be conveyed to a pharmacy?
I.   As a written prescription
II.   By fax
III.   By e-mail
(A) I only   (B) III only   (C) I & II only
(D) II & III only   (E) I, II, & III

39.   Under which of the following conditions may a pharmaceutical sales representative distribute samples of a prescription drug product?
I.   Upon written request from a community pharmacy
II.   Upon written request from a hospital pharmacy
III.   Upon written request from a physician
(A) I only   (B) III only   (C) I & II only
(D) II & III only   (E) I, II, & III

40. Benzadrex Inhalers are an example of a product
classified as
(A) Schedule II   (B) Schedule III   (C) Schedule IV
(D) ScheduleV   (E) Noncontrolled

41. The expiration date on a commercial pharmaceutical
product is July 2008. The actual date that this product
will be considered expired will be after:
(A) June 30th   (B) July 1st   (C) July 15th
(D) July 31st   (E) August 1st

42. A patient presents a prescription for sixty Empirin
w/codeine tablets No.4 to his local pharmacy and
indicates that he would only like to get 30 of the tablets
now and will return for the other 30 in a week if the
medication agrees with him. The pharmacist
should
(A)   call the prescriber to get permission to dispense 30
(B)   dispense 30 tablets as requested by the patient.
(C)   advise the patient that the full 60 tablets must
      be supplied at one time.
(D)   fill the prescription as requested by the patient
      but advise the patient that the balance must be
      picked up within 72 hours.
(E)   dispense 30 tablets of Empirin w/codeine No. 2
      tablets.

43. Prescriptions written for Accutane may not exceed
I.   a quantity of 30 capsules
II. a one month supply
III. six refills of one month quantities
(A) I only   (B) III only   (C) I & II only
(D) II & III only (E) I, II, & III

44.   Which of the following is/are true regarding the sale of codeine-containing schedule V cough medicine without a prescription?
I.   Only a pharmacist may dispense the product to the consumer.
II.   A non-pharmacist may "ring-up" the sale and collect payment for the product.
III.   Not more than 120 mL or 24 dosage units of this product may be sold to the same purchaser in any 7-day period.
(A) I only   (B) III only   (C) I & II only
(D) II & III only   (E) I, II, & III

45.   Which dosage forms of secobarbital must be ordered using a DEA Form 222?
I.   Capsule
II.   Injectable
III.   Suppository
(A) I only   (B) III only   (C) I & II only
(D) II & III only   (E) I, II, & III

46.   Davis Labs is the first to place a new drug product on the market. This product would be described in the Orange Book as:
I.   a reference drug product
II.   B rated
III.   AB rated
(A) I only   (B) III only   (C) I & II only
(D) II & III only   (E) I, II, & III

47.   Major objectives for developing a formulary include:
I.   reduce drug inventory
II.   allow therapeutic substitution
III.   give prescribers a greater latitude of drug selection
(A) I only   (B) III only   (C) I & II only
(D) II & III only   (E) I, II, & III

48. A pharmacist who does not receive a registration renewal form from DEA within 45 days before the expiration of his/her registration must notify
I.   his/her state's board of pharmacy
II.   the regional FDA office
III.   the DEA in writing and request renewal forms
(A) I only   (B) III only   (C) I & II only
(D) II & III only   (E) I, II, & III

49. Which of the following reference book(s) is(are) legal documents recognized by the federal government?
I.   *Remington's Pharmaceutical Sciences*
II.   *Homeopathic Pharmacopeia of the U.S.*
III.   *USP/NF*
(A) I only   (B) III only   (C) I & II only
(D) II & III only   (E) I, II, & III

50. Which one of the following is MOST important to consider in determining whether a community pharmacy is required to meet HIPAA regulations?
(A) The prescription volume is greater than 20,000 per year.
(B) The store's annual income is greater than 1 million dollars.
(C) The pharmacy accepts Medicaid prescriptions.
(D) Identifiable patient health information is transferred electronically.
(E) The pharmacy has more than 10 employees.

51. Which of the following sublingual tablets do NOT have to be dispensed in child-resistant containers?
I.   Nitroglycerin
II.   Nitrostat
III.   Isordil
(A) I only   (B) III only   (C) I & II only
(D) II & III only   (E) I, II, & III

52. Which of the following drug products may be purchased by a pharmacy WITHOUT the use of a DEA Form 222?
I.   Lorcet Tablets
II.   Stadol
III.   Mepergan Injection

(A) I only   (B) III only   (C) I & II only
(D) II & III only   (E) I, II, & III

53.   Which of the following products are exempt from the
        FDA regulations concerning expiration dating?
        I.   USP/NF drug products
        II.   dietary supplements
        III.   vitamins
        (A) I only   (B) III only   (C) I & II only
        (D) II & III only   (E) I, II, & III

54.   Guidelines for determining the expiration date for
        repackaging of a drug product by a pharmacy includes:
        I.   not more than the expiration date on the original
                package
        II.   not more than one year from the date of
                packaging
        III.   one-half of the time remaining on the original
                package
        (A) I only   (B) III only   (C) I & II only
        (D) II & III only   (E) I, II, & III

55.   A physician who is a resident in a hospital and does
        not have a DEA registration number
        (A)   may not prescribe controlled substances.
        (B)   may only prescribe controlled substances for
                outpatients.
        (C)   may prescribe controlled substances using the
                hospital DEA number plus an assigned suffix.
        (D)   may prescribe controlled substances only in
                Schedule III-V.
        (E)   may prescribe only for inpatients.

56. If a specific lot of a pharmaceutical company's tablets fails to meet the expected expiration dating, the lot may be considered to be:
    - (A) adulterated
    - (B) unstable
    - (C) misbranded
    - (D) a class III recall
    - (E) a felony

57. What is the longest "beyond use" expiration date that a pharmacist may place on a prescription container if the original drug container label states "expiration date 1/08"? Assume the pharmacist fills the prescription on January 2, 2005.
    - (A) 7/2/05   (B) 1/2/06   (C) 7/2/06
    - (D) 1/1/08   (E) 1/31/08

58. Who is authorized to designate the "official" name for a new drug?
    - (A) Director of the FDA
    - (B) Executive Director of APHA
    - (C) Director of HCFA
    - (D) Secretary of HHS
    - (E) U.S. Congress

59. Which of the following activities are considered illegal if an individual is receiving prescription drugs by mail from a Canadian pharmacy?
    - I.   Splitting the drug supply with his neighbor who also has a prescription
    - II. Receiving a six months supply of the drug
    - III. Having the drug mailed directly to his home rather than to his physician
    - (A) I only   (B) III only   (C) I & II only
    - (D) II & III only   (E) I, II, & III

60. The federal act that specifically limits the reimportation of drug products that were previously exported by a pharmaceutical manufacturer is the:

(A)   FD & C Act of 1938
(B)   Durham-Humphrey Act
(C)   Prescription Drug Marketing Act of 1987
(D)   DSHEA
(E)   Kefauver-Harris Amendment of 1962

61.   A pharmacist may fill prescriptions for and mail which of the following drugs through the US Postal Service?
   I.   Schedule II non-narcotics
   II.   Benzodiazepines
   III.   Schedule II narcotics
   (A) I only   (B) III only   (C) I & II only
   (D) II & III only   (E) I, II, & III

62.   Which of the following actions are appropriate when mailing a narcotic drug filled using a valid prescripttion?
   I.   Package the drug container in a plain paper outer wrapping
   II.   Place the warning: "Narcotic, do not open while in transit" on the outer wrapping
   III.   Place a fictitious return address on the outer wrapping.
   (A) I only   (B) III only   (C) I & II only
   (D) II & III only   (E) I, II, & III

63.   Labels on cosmetic packages must have ingredients listed:
   (A) in descending order of concentration
   (B) ascending order of concentration
   (C) alphabetically
   (D) any random order
   (E) with the most active listed first

64. Samples of prescription drugs received from pharmaceutical companies may be
(A) sold through community pharmacies
(B) dispensed from a hospital pharmacy for inpatients
(C) dispensed from a hospital to outpatients
(D) given to patients by a prescriber
(E) traded to another pharmacy for other drugs

65. A pharmacy clinician is preparing a research paper which describes the side effects of LMW heparins in 20 of her patients. Which of the following patient information must be removed from the paper before submission for publication?
I. home address   II. social security number   III. age
(A) I only   (B) III only   (C) I & II only
(D) II & III only   (E) I, II, & III

66. Proposed regulations from the FDA are first published in the:
(A) Congressional Record   (B) Federal Register
(C) New York Times and Wall Street Journal
(D) USP/NF   (E) Supplements of the USP/NF

67. A physician telephones a pharmacy and prescribes 40 Percodan tablets, 1 TID. Which of the following is/are true?
I.   It may only be dispensed in an emergency.
II.   A written "cover" prescription must be received before the pharmacist may dispense the medication.
III. Not more than a 7-day supply may be prescribed orally.
(A) I only   (B) III only   (C) I & II only
(D) II & III only (E) I, II, & III

68. Which of the following controlled drugs may a pharmacist mail through the US Postal Service?
I.   Schedule II's
II.   Schedule III's
III. Schedule IV's
(A) I only   (B) III only   (C) I & II only
(D) II & III only (E) I, II, & III

69.   A community pharmacy develops and prepares
        batches of 5,000 sustained release capsules similar to
        a commercially available product but at a lower price.
        The pharmacy may be cited for this activity based
        upon:
        I.   The capsule formula may be considered a
              new drug
        II.   The preparation of 5,000 capsules may be
              considered manufacturing.
        III. The failure to following GMPs.
        (A) I only   (B) III only   (C) I & II only
        (D) II & III only   (E) I, II, & III

70.   A pharmacy that compounds large numbers of
        prescriptions may be cited by the FDA if its volume
        of prescriptions being sent to out-of-state is in excess
        of ____ %.
        (A) 25   (B) 5   (C) 40
        (D) 10   (E) 75

71.   A patient presents a prescription for MS Contin
        30mg tablets # 60 to his local pharmacy and
        indicates that he would only like to get 30 of the
        tablets now and will return for the other 30 in a week
        if the medication agrees with him. The pharmacist
        should
        (A)   call the prescriber to get permission to dispense
                30.
        (B)   dispense 30 tablets as requested by the patient.
        (C)   advise the patient that the full 60 tablets must
                be supplied at one time.
        (D)   fill the prescription as requested by the patient
                but advise the patient that the balance must be
                picked up within 72 hours.
        (E)   dispense 30 tablets of the 60 mg strength of MS
                Contin.

72.   Which of the following protocols must a hospital phar-
        macy follow in order to possess pharmaceutical manu-
        facturer's drug samples?
        I.   The hospital must be registered as a drug
                wholesaler.
        II.   The hospital must store the samples separate
                from the regular stock.
        III.   A licensed practitioner must have requested the
                samples from the company.
        (A) I only   (B) III only   (C) I & II only
        (D) II & III only   (E) I, II, & III

73.   The names of which of the following ingredients are
        required to be included on the labels of pharmaceutical
        products?
        I.   antimicrobial preservatives
        II.   coloring agents
        III.   flavoring oils
        (A) I only   (B) III only   (C) I & II only
        (D) II & III only   (E) I, II, & III

74.   Which one of the following is the correct format for the
        listing of ingredients on a product label?
        (A)   The additives and active ingredients intermixed
                but in alphabetical sequence.
        (B)   Additives and active ingredients intermixed but
                ranked by decreasing concentrations.
        (C)   Additives and active ingredients intermixed but
                ranked by increasing concentrations.
        (D)   Additives listed separately from the active
                ingredients.
        (E)   Additives listed separately by decreasing
                concentrations.

75.   When listing an ingredient on a product label, all of the
        following references may be used by manufacturers as
        primary sources for names EXCEPT.
        (A) CTFA Cosmetic Ingredient Dictionary
        (B) Facts and Comparisons
        (C) Food Chemicals Codex
        (D) USAN
        (E) USP Dictionary of Drug Names

76.   Which one of the following reference sources is the first choice when a manufacturer is determining the preferred name of an additive for a product label?
(A) CTFA Cosmetic Ingredient Dictionary
(B) Food Chemicals Codex
(C) USAN
(D) USP Dictionary of Drug Names
(E) USP/NF

77.   According to Federal regulations, a color additive may not be added to which one of the following dosage forms?
(A) capsules   (B) parenteral solutions   (C) syrups
(D) tablets   (E) topical lotions

78.   Which of the following volumes of the USP/DI contains significant information concerning the bio-equivalence of drug products?
I.   Volume I
II.   Volume II
III. Volume III
(A) I only   (B) III only   (C) I & II only
(D) II & III only   (E) I, II, & III

79.   The major objective of the Orange Book is to compare drug products that are
I.   multisourced
II.   most economical
III. different dosage forms
(A) I only   (B) III only   (C) I & II only
(D) II & III only   (E) I, II, & III

80. Which of the following was the first to require that pharmaceutical manufacturers prove the safety of prescription drugs before marketing?
(A)   Durham-Humphrey Amendment (1951)
(B)   F D & C Act of 1938
(C)   Kefauver-Harris Amendment of 1962
(D)   Prescription Drug Marketing Act of 1987
(E)   Pure Food and Drug Act of 1906

81. Which of the following designations indicate that drug products of the same strength and dosage form may be interchangeable?
I.   BC
II.   AB
III. A
(A) I only   (B) III only   (C) I & II only
(D) II & III only   (E) I, II, & III

82. The Electronic Orange Book uses the symbol "RLD", in a series of similar drug products to indicate:
(A)   the drug products that have not been assessed
(B)   that there is no bioequivalence problem
(C)   the drug product that is preferred by most pharmacists for substitution
(D)   the least expensive drug product
(E)   the product used as reference standard

83. Drug products with which of the following codes may be substituted for one another?
I.   A
II.   AB
III. B
(A) I only   (B) III only   (C) I & II only
(D) II & III only   (E) I, II, & III

84. Original packages of nitroglycerin that are exempt from the requirements of the Poison Prevention Packaging Act include:
I.   oral tablets
II.   ointments
III. SL tablets

(A) I only   (B) III only   (C) I & II only
(D) II & III only   (E) I, II, & III

85.   Which one of the following dosage forms is least
      likely to present bioequivalence problems?
      (A) capsule   (B) IV solution   (C) suspension
      (D) transdermal patch   (E) tablet

86.   Certain drug products are exempt from the requirements
      of therapeutic equivalence because of:
      I.   their high therapeutic index
      II.   their use in chemotherapy
      III. the grandfather clause
      (A) I only   (B) III only   (C) I & II only
      (D) II & III only   (E) I, II, & III

87.   Which of the following commercial products intended
      for oral intake need identification codes on the
      individual units?
      I.   Nonprescription tablets
      II.   Prescription tablets
      III. Prescription capsules dosage forms
      (A) I only   (B) III only   (C) I & II only
      (D) II & III only   (E) I, II, & III

88.   Which of the following employees may administer or
      dispense drugs to patients as part of a narcotic treatment
      program?
      I.   Pharmacists
      II.   Registered nurses
      III. Licensed practical nurses
      (A) I only   (B) III only   (C) I & II only
      (D) II & III only   (E) I, II, & III

89.   Which of the following reference sources contain
      significant information concerning the bioequivalence of
      drug products?

I. USP/NF
II. USP/DI
III. Orange Book
(A) I only   (B) III only   (C) I & II only
(D) II & III only (E) I, II, & III

90. Permission to not use a child-resistant closure on a prescription may be granted by the
I. pharmacist
II. prescriber
III. patient
(A) I only   (B) III only   (C) I & II only
(D) II & III only (E) I, II, & III

91. Enforcement of the PPPA is basically under the jurisdiction of the:
(A)   Food and Drug Administration (FDA)
(B)   Federal Trade Commission (FTC)
(C)   Consumer Product Safety Commission (CPSC)
(D)   US Justice Department
(E)   Health Care Financing Administration (HCFA)

92. The term used in the HIPAA privacy rules to describe the removal of patient identifying information when discussing a specific clinical case in public is:
(A) debriefing   (B) de-indentification
(C) document erasure   (D) depersonalization
(E) anti-terrorist protection

93. Packaging for nonprescription products that is designed to prevent the addition of foreign material into the final product is best described as being:
(A) tamper-evident   (B) tamper-proof
(C) tamper-resistant   (D) hermetically sealed
(E) air-tight

94.   The purchasing agent of your hospital suggests that the hospital purchase a two-year's supply of a popular antibiotic at a special price. Which of the following are legal activities?
I.   purchase of that quantity of the antibiotic
II.   sell a portion of the antibiotic to another area hospital
III.   sell a portion of the antibiotic to a community pharmacy
(A) I only   (B) III only   (C) I & II only
(D) II & III only   (E) I, II, & III

95.   Uses for tax-free alcohol purchased by a hospital may include:
I.   incorporation into formulas for inpatient orders
II.   incorporation into prescriptions for recently discharged patients
III.   selling of small amounts to independent pharmacies based upon their immediate prescription needs
(A) I only   (B) III only   (C) I & II only
(D) II & III only   (E) I, II, & III

96.   The classification of drugs into controlled substance schedules by the federal government is based upon the drug's
I.   toxicity
II.   therapeutic index
III.   potential for abuse and dependence
(A) I only   (B) III only   (C) I & II only
(D) II & III only   (E) I, II, & III

97.   A neighboring community pharmacy requests Alcohol USP/NF from your hospital pharmacy, which has tax-free alcohol. Under what circumstances may you supply the alcohol?

(A)   It is never permissible
(B)   Limiting your sale to not more than one pint
(C)   By making a simple loan of the alcohol
(D)   Any circumstances are permissible
(E)   By charging the pharmacy the purchase
        price plus the alcohol tax

98.   The maximum volume of Ipecac Syrup that may be
        sold without a prescription is:
        (A) 15 mL (B) 120mL (C) 60 mL (D) 30 mL
        (E) 240 mL

99.   Under which of the following circumstances may Ipecac
        Syrup be sold without a prescription?
        I.   For future potential use during accidental poisoning.
        II.   Only if the household does not have small
              Children.
        III. For limited use in a weight-loss program.
        (A) I only   (B) III only   (C) I & II only
        (D) II & III only   (E) I, II, & III

100.   The label of a bottle of Ipecac Syrup sold OTC for
        accidental poisoning must:
        I.   have its warnings printed in red ink.
        II.   contain the telephone number of the regional
              poison control center.
        III. state that the appropriate dose is the entire
              bottle followed by a full glass of water.
        (A) I only   (B) III only   (C) I & II only
        (D) II & III only   (E) I, II, & III

101.   An orphan drug is one that has
        (A)   been removed from the market because of
                toxicity
        (B)   has been discontinued because of poor sales
        (C)   provided special economic incentives for the
                manufacturer
        (D)   has a low therapeutic index
        (E)   has been developed and imported from a foreign
                country

102.   Pharmacists may transfer prescription information on a one-time basis for the purpose of dispensing a refill for which of the following drug products?
I.   Lomotil tablets
II.   Dalmane capsules
III. Tylenol w/codeine capsules
(A) I only   (B) III only   (C) I & II only
(D) II & III only   (E) I, II, & III

103.   Which one of the following organizations is directly responsible for Medicare programs?
(A) FDA   (B) HCFA   (C) HMO
(D) JCAHO   (E) AARP

104.   A product that contains 60 mg of codeine and 325mg of acetaminophen is most likely to be classified as
(A) Schedule II   (B) Schedule III   (C) Schedule IV
(D) ScheduleV   (E) Noncontrolled

105.   Prescription drug package inserts include all of the following types of information EXCEPT:
(A)   adverse reactions
(B)   contraindications
(C)   symptoms and treatment of overdosing
(D)   AWP's
(E)   date of most recent revision of the labeling

106.   Which one of the following types of information found in the prescription drug package insert is most critical in determining whether to dispense a certain drug to a specific patient?
(A)   adverse reactions
(B)   contraindications
(C)   cautions
(D)   warnings
(E)   indications

107. When refilling a prescription that requires a child-resistant container, the pharmacist must always replace which of the following?
     I.   The plastic closure
     II. The plastic container
     III. The glass container
     (A) I only   (B) III only   (C) I & II only
     (D) II & III only   (E) I, II, & III

108. Which of the following categories of pregnancy warnings is the most severe?
     (A)   Category A
     (B)   Category D
     (C)   Category III
     (D)   Category X
     (E)   Category NR

109. Under which one of the following circumstances may a pharmacist refuse to fill a prescription?
     (A)   The quantity of the controlled drug has been changed.
     (B)   The pharmacist does not know the patient.
     (C)   The patient is an alcoholic.
     (D)   The prescription was written a week ago.
     (E)   The prescriber is from another city.

110. According to the present DSHEA, an herbal product such as Saw Palmetto may be labeled to state:
     (A)   cures prostatitis
     (B)   help treat prostatitis
     (C)   for the prostate
     (D)   helps in prevention of prostate cancer
     (E)   will return the prostate to normal size

111. Every new drug placed on the market will have a designated
     I.   generic name
     II. tradename
     III. brandname
     (A) I only   (B) III only   (C) I & II only
     (D) II & III only   (E) I, II, & III

112. In which of the following locations would you NOT
      find pharmaceutical manufacturer's drug samples?
      I.   hospital pharmacy
      II.   physician's office
      III. chain or community pharmacy
      (A) I only   (B) III only   (C) I & II only
      (D) II & III only   (E) I, II, & III

113. What number is given to the clinical trial phase that
      consists of post-marketing surveillance of a drug that
      was recently introduced onto the market?
      (A) 1   (B) 2   (C) 3   (D) 4   (E) 5

114. With respect to pregnancy warnings, category D
      indicates that the drug
      (A)   is safe for 98% of all females during pregnancy.
      (B)   should not be used during the first trimester.
      (C)   should be administered only if the potential
             benefits are acceptable despite the potential
             risks.
      (D)   should not be used during the pregnancy.
      (E)   does not pose any danger to either the mother
             or fetus.

115. Which one of the following laws first required the
      statement "Caution: Federal law prohibits dispensing
      without a prescription" on drug product packaging?
      (A)   Durham-Humphrey Amendment
      (B)   FD & C Act of 1938
      (C)   Kefauver-Harris Amendment
      (D)   Prescription Drug Marketing Act
      (E)   Pure Food and Drug Act of 1906

116. DEA registration numbers that are assigned to mid-level
      practioners generally begin with which of the following
      letters?
      (A) A   (B) B   (C) M
      (D) L   (E) X

117. A product that contains not more than 1.8 g of codeine per 100 mL is considered to be in Schedule
(A) I   (B) II   (C) III
(D) IV   (E) V

118. Dronabinol is a Schedule II controlled substance that is related most closely to
(A) cocaine   (B) morphine   (C) LSD
(D) marijuana   (E) methylphenidate

119. Which of the following is true of Schedule V substances?
  I. They all contain codeine.
  II. When they are dispensed by the pharmacist, the federal transfer warning must be on the container labeling..
  III. Some states may permit sale of these products without a prescription.
(A) I only   (B) III only   (C) I & II only
(D) II & III only   (E) I, II, & III

120. Hospital inpatients receiving oral estrogen therapy must receive patient package inserts:
(A) every day
(B) only with the first dose
(C) at least every 30 days
(D) at least every 7 days
(E) only at the first dose and when being discharged

121. Which one of the following acronyms is most closely associated with health care reimbursement?
(A) DEA   (B) DRG   (C) GMP
(D) JCAHO   (E) PPI

122. Hospitalized patients that are part of a comprehensive narcotic treatment program may receive methadone doses by which of the following routes?
  I. Oral
  II. Parenteral
  III. Transdermal

(A) I only   (B) III only   (C) I & II only
(D) II & III only   (E) I, II, & III

123. Two generic companies manufacture a specific drug in several dosage forms. Which one of the dosage forms is MOST likely to present problems with bioequivalence?
(A)   aerosol
(B)   capsule
(C)   oral solution
(D)   parenteral solution
(E)   tablet

124. Which government body is responsible for funding and overseeing state Medicaid programs?
(A) DHHS   (B) FDA   (C) HCFA
(D) NABP   (E) USP/NF

125. The National Drug Code (NDC) consists of a series of
(A)   letters only
(B)   letters and numbers
(C)   numbers only
(D)   numbers and symbols
(E)   symbols only

126. The first series of digits in the NDC for a drug product represents the:
(A)   drug name
(B)   drug strength
(C)   manufacturer
(D)   package size
(E)   therapeutic use

127. The acronym, DUR, is most closely associated with which of the following?
(A) Drug clinical trials
(B) Medicare reimbursement
(C) MedWatch
(D) Drug nomenclature
(E) Patient counseling

128. Schedule III, IV, or V controlled substances may be refilled
I. not more than 6 times
II. not more than for a 6 month period
III. only if authorized by the prescriber
(A) I only   (B) III only   (C) I & II only
(D) II & III only   (E) I, II, & III

129. The drug patent of an innovator company has expired. Which one of the following must a second drug company submit to place a generic form of the drug product onto the market?
(A) Abbreviated new drug application
(B) Investigational new drug application
(C) New drug application
(D) Generic drug application
(E) Supplemental new drug application

130. Hospitals that plan on using large quantities of tax-free grain alcohol should obtain which one of the following forms?
(A) ATF 11   (B) ATF 222   (C) ATF 1447
(D) DEA 222   (E) DEA 1447

131. Oral authorization for additional refills on a schedule III prescription are acceptable as long as
 I. the total quantity authorized does not exceed five refills within a six-month period from the date of issue of the original prescription.
 II. the quantity of each additional refill authorized is not greater than the quantity authorized for the initial filling of the prescription.
 III. the pharmacist gets a "cover" prescription from the prescriber within 7 days of the oral authorization.
 (A) I only   (B) III only   (C) I & II only
 (D) II & III only   (E) I, II, & III

132. The Poison Prevention Packaging Act (PPPA) is intended to protect
 I. young children
 II. geriatric patients
 III. potentially suicidal patients
 (A) I only   (B) III only   (C) I & II only
 (D) II & III only   (E) I, II, & III

133. Which of the following must be imprinted on each commercial oral tablet?
 (A)   Company name
 (B)   Name and strength of the drug
 (C)   A code identifying each of the above
 (D)   An expiration date
 (E)   Date of manufacturing

134. Which one of the following actions is permissible in a hospital that has tax-free alcohol?
 (A)   dispensing to inpatients in the form of a tonic
 (B)   loan pint quantities to community pharmacies
 (C)   loan pint quantities to other hospitals
 (D)   sell pint quantities to community pharmacies
 (E)   sell pint quantities to physician offices

135. The main responsibility for oversight of prescription drug advertising rests with the
(A) FDA   (B) FTC   (C) HCFA
(D) DEA   (E) USP/NF

136. A drug product consisting of tablets may be declared adulterated for all of the following reasons EXCEPT:
(A)   active drug has undergone partial decomposition
(B)   contains an unapproved color additive
(C)   does not indicate number of tablets present
(D)   inactive ingredient has undergone partial decomposition
(E)   manufactured in a plant that fails to meet GMP's

137. Based upon the Federal Anti-drug Abuse Act of 1988, a pharmacy employee who is convicted of criminal possession of illegal drugs must:
(A)   inform his/her employer within 5 days of the conviction
(B)   inform his/her employer within one year of the conviction
(C)   volunteer to enter a drug rehabilitation program
(D)   volunteer to perform at least 1000 hours of community service
(E)   resign his/her position from a pharmacy

138. Excipients included in pharmaceutical dosage forms are usually found on which of the following lists?
(A) DSHEA   (B) GRAS   (C) HPLC
(D) Top 200   (E) UPS

139. Which one of the following pieces of information is NOT encoded into a drug product's NDC?
(A)   drug name
(B)   manufacturer
(C)   product's expiration date
(D)   package size
(E)   strength of a tablet

140. Mr. Hess has not picked up a prescription that was filled
     last week. Which of the following actions is (are) legal
     for the pharmacist to take?
     I.   call the patient at home and leave a message with his
          son
     II. call the patient and leave a message on his home
          answering machine.
     III. send an E-Mail to the patient's web site
     (A) I only   (B) III only   (C) I & II only
     (D) II & III only   (E) I, II, & III

141. A drug product consisting of tablets may be declared
     misbranded under all of the following guidelines
     EXCEPT:
     (A)   does not meet assay limits
     (B)   does not indicate number of tablets present
     (C)   official names of certain ingredients not used
     (D)   name and location of manufacturer is missing
     (E)   portion of the label is misleading

142. Which form must a community pharmacy use to
     purchase grain alcohol for compounding?
     (A) ATF 11   (B) ATF 222   (C) DEA 222
     (D) DEA 23a   (E) FDA 23a

143. The Marketing Act of 1987 guarantees a company
     that discovers, patents, and develops a new drug ex-
     clusive marketing rights for up to:
     (A) 20 years   (B) 10 years   (C) 17 years
     (D) 50 years   (E) 100 years

144. When a Schedule II prescription is partially filled for
     a LTCF patient

I.   the prescription is valid not more than 60 days from the issue date.

II. the pharmacist must write "LTCF patient" on the prescription.

III. the total quantity dispensed cannot exceed 100 dosage units.

(A) I only   (B) III only   (C) I & II only

(D) II & III only (E) I, II, & III

145.   Which of the following are exempt from registration under the Controlled Substance Act?

I.   A U.S. Army physician

II. A U.S. Public Health Service physician

III. A foreign-trained physician

(A) I only   (B) III only   (C) I & II only

(D) II & III only (E) I, II, & III

146.   The statement "Caution: Federal law prohibits the transfer of this drug to any person other than the patient for whom it was prescribed" is not required for

I.   controlled substances dispensed for use in "blinded" clinical investigations.

II. dispensing Schedule V drugs.

III. dispensing controlled substances to be administered to a patient in an institution.

(A) I only   (B) III only   (C) I & II only

(D) II & III only (E) I, II, & III

147.   The total number of digits in the NDC numbers present on a pharmaceutical package may be:

(A) 2 or 3   (B) 5 or 6   (C) 8 or 9

(D) 10 or 11   (E) 15 to 16

148.   Which of the following is true about DEA Form 222?

I.   If it contains incorrect information the supplier may correct it and initial the correction.

II. If an order cannot be filled by a supplier the form must be returned to the purchaser.

III. If any forms are lost, the loss must be reported to DEA.

(A) I only   (B) III only   (C) I & II only
(D) II & III only   (E) I, II, & III

149.   A hospital that has two 55-gallon drums of tax-free grain alcohol must:
       (A)   maintain a running inventory of the volume
       (B)   inventory the stock every month
       (C)   inventory the stock every 6 months
       (D)   report the amount remaining to the ATF every six months
       (E)   take a year-end inventory

150.   The term "Grandfathered" refers to drugs that were marketed before
       (A)   FD & C Act of 1938
       (B)   Durham-Humphrey Act
       (C)   DSHEA
       (D)   Kefauver-Harris Amendment of 1962
       (E)   Poison Prevention Act

151.   A statement that a specific OTC product has a tamper-evident feature may be placed in any of the following locations EXCEPT on the:
       (A)   closure
       (B)   front of the package
       (C)   back of the package
       (D)   on the tamper-evident device
       (E)   under the product name

152.   Which of the following drug products must be purchased using a DEA Form 222?
       I.   Levoprome
       II. Demerol
       III. Duragesic-50
       (A) I only   (B) III only   (C) I & II only
       (D) II & III only   (E) I, II, & III

153. Which of the following agents is an anabolic steroid?
    I. nandrolone
    II. fluticasone
    III. hydrocortisone
    (A) I only   (B) III only   (C) I & II only
    (D) II & III only   (E) I, II, & III

154. "Grandfathered" drugs are
    (A)   found in the Orange Book as Code A only.
    (B)   found in the Orange Book as Code B only.
    (C)   found in the Orange Book as Code AB only.
    (D)   to be prescribed only by generic name.
    (E)   often not listed in the Orange Book.

155. A pharmacy that compounds many prescriptions may be cited by the FDA if the volume of its prescriptions being sent to out-of-state is in excess of _____ %.
    (A) 2   (B) 5   (C) 10
    (D) 20   (E) 50

156. Into how many segments is the NDC number on a pharmaceutical package divided?
    (A) 2   (B) 3   (C) 4
    (D) 5   (E) greater than 5

157. The first phase of a clinical trial, which evaluates the efficacy of the drug in treating a specific disease, is:
    (A) phase I   (B) phase II   (C) phase III
    (D) phase IV   (E) phase V

158. Under which of the following conditions may practitioners of "Traditional Chinese Medicine" sell ephedra-containing products?
    (A) The level of ephedra is less than 1 mg per dose.
    (B) Only a 10 day supply of product is sold.
    (C) The label does not indicate that the product is a dietary supplement.
    (D) A prescription is issued for the product.
    (E) Sales are not legal

159. A customer enters your pharmacy and requests 25 x 260 mg quinine tablets. Which of the following responses by the pharmacist would be appropriate?
I.   Quinine tablets can no longer be sold over-the-counter.
II.   OTC quinine is considered to be unsafe for the prevention of malaria.
III. OTC quinine is considered ineffective for the treatment of nocturnal leg cramps.
(A) I only   (B) III only   (C) I & II only
(D) II & III only   (E) I, II, & III

160. Which of the following are mid-level practitioners?
I.   Nurse Practitioners
II.   Nurse Midwives
III. Podiatrists
(A) I only   (B) III only   (C) I & II only
(D) II & III only   (E) I, II, & III

161. Under which of the following circumstances may Ipecac Syrup be sold without a prescription?
I.   for future potential use during accidental poisoning
II.   only if the household does not have small children
III. if the purchaser signs a pharmacy log book for the sale
(A) I only   (B) III only   (C) I & II only
(D) II & III only   (E) I, II, & III

162. Which of the following forms are used to apply for a new DEA registration for a community pharmacy?
I.   Form 222
II.   Form 222a
III. Form 224
(A) I only   (B) III only   (C) I & II only
(D) II & III only   (E) I, II, & III

163. Short-term detoxification treatment is defined as treatment that does not exceed
(A) 24 hours   (B) 7 days   (C) 30 days
(D) 90 days   (E) 180 days

164. Which of the following clinical trial stages is conducted exclusively in healthy humans?
(A) phase I   (B) phase II   (C) phase III
(D) phase IV   (E) phase I and II

165. Which of the following drugs are considered to be "Basic Class" drugs under the Controlled Substances Act?
I.   dextroamphetamine
II.   codeine
III. phenobarbital
(A) I only   (B) III only   (C) I & II only
(D) II & III only   (E) I, II, & III

166. Which one of the following incentives is used to encourage pharmaceutical companies to conduct studies of their drugs in the pediatric population?
(A)   grants of money from the FDA
(B)   extension of patent protection
(C)   refunds of income tax
(D)   tax credits for subsequent years
(E)   letter of commendation from the President

167. A policeman visits your pharmacy and informs you that he has arrested an individual suspected of writing a prescription using a fictitious doctor's information. Since the prescription was filled in your pharmacy, the officer requests the original prescription as evidence. Which of the following statements relating to this incidence is (are) correct?
I.   You should give him the prescription if he gives you a written receipt.
II   Legally, the described prescription is not a forged prescription.
III. You are not obligated to give him the prescription.

(A) I only   (B) III only   (C) I & II only
(D) II & III only   (E) I, II, & III

168.   Orphan drugs are drugs that are intended for the
       (A)   treatment of rare diseases
       (B)   chemically dissimilar to any other marketed
               drug moiety
       (C)   intended for use in children under the age of 16
       (D)   intended for use in children under the age of 5
       (E)   administered to children without the permission
               of their parents

169.   Labels of commercial drug products that are intended for
       electrolyte replacement must contain the concentration
       expressed in terms of:
       I.   weight or concentration
       II.   milliequivalents
       III. millimoles
       (A) I only   (B) III only   (C) I & II only
       (D) II & III only   (E) I, II, & III

170.   Which of the following are Schedule II controlled
       substances?
       I.   sufentanyl
       II.   psilocyn
       III. chloral hydrate
       (A) I only   (B) III only   (C) I & II only
       (D) II & III only   (E) I, II, & III

171.   Phenobarbital is a drug that is classified as a(n)
       (A) Schedule III drug   (B) Schedule IV drug
       (C) Schedule V drug   (D) non-controlled drug
       (E) OTC drug

172. All of the following drugs fall into the category of "Grandfathered Drugs" EXCEPT:
 (A) ampicillin
 (B) ephedrine
 (C) epinephrine
 (D) phenobarbital
 (E) thyroid

173. Percogesic is an example of a product that is
 (A) in Schedule II   (B) in Schedule III
 (C) in Schedule IV   (D) in Schedule V
 (E) not a controlled substance

174. How often must a pharmacy have a patient sign a new notice that he/she has been informed of the pharmacy's privacy practices under HIPAA requirements?
 (A) Every time a new prescription is filled
 (B) Every time a refill is dispensed
 (C) Every 6 months
 (D) Every year
 (E) No requirements are specified by HIPAA

175. The original portion of the Form 222 is eventually kept on file by the
 (A) DEA   (B) purchaser   (C) FDA
 (D) supplier   (E) prescriber

176. Copy 3 of DEA Form 222 is eventually kept by the
 (A) DEA   (B) supplier   (C) purchaser
 (D) prescriber (E) FDA

177. Which of the following barbiturates are classified as Schedule II controlled substances?
 I. amobarbital
 II. pentobarbital
 III. butabarbital
 (A) I only   (B) III only   (C) I & II only
 (D) II & III only (E) I, II, & III

178.   Which of the following is true about DEA Form 222?
I.   It may be used by any pharmacy in the same chain
II.   It may be partially filled by the supplier
III.   A physician may use it to order Schedule II controlled substances
(A) I only   (B) III only   (C) I & II only
(D) II & III only   (E) I, II, & III

179.   Which of the following products are Schedule III controlled substances?
I.   Demerol tablets
II.   Empirin with Codeine #3
III.   Tylenol with Codeine #1
(A) I only   (B) III only   (C) I & II only
(D) II & III only   (E) I, II, & III

180.   A pharmaceutical manufacturer requests from a community pharmacy the names and addresses of patients receiving the company's antidepressant so that a special discount coupons may be provided for future prescriptions . This scenario is probably in violation of which of the following laws?
(A) DSHEA
(B) FDA Modernization Act of 1997
(C) HIPAA
(D) OBRA 90
(E) Sherman Antitrust Act

181.   A filled DEA Form 222 must be kept by the
I.   supplier for 2 years
II.   purchaser for 3 years
III.   DEA for 10 years
(A) I only   (B) III only   (C) I & II only
(D) II & III only   (E) I, II, & III

182. Which of the following is true of DEA Form 222?
    I.   It is used to order Schedule II controlled substances
    II. Only one product may be ordered on each line of the form
    III. May be used to order syringes and hypodermic needles.
    (A) I only   (B) III only   (C) I & II only
    (D) II & III only   (E) I, II, & III

183. Controlled substances prescriptions may be issued by prescribers
    I.   to obtain controlled substances for dispensing in their office
    II. to prescribe drugs to be used by a patient for narcotic detoxification
    III to prescribe controlled substances for a patient with chronic pain.
    (A) I only   (B) III only   (C) I & II only
    (D) II & III only   (E) I, II, & III

184. Controlled substance prescriptions
    I.   may be written by typewriter (except for the prescriber's signature).
    II. must have the name of the physician printed, stamped, typed, or hand-printed on it.
    III. may be prepared by an agent of the prescriber for the prescriber's signature
    (A) I only   (B) III only   (C) I & II only
    (D) II & III only   (E) I, II, & III

185. Which of the following are Schedule IV controlled substances?
    I.   flurazepam
    II. halazepam
    III. zolpidem
    (A) I only   (B) III only   (C) I & II only
    (D) II & III only   (E) I, II, & III

186.   Any physician is permitted to
    I.   prescribe drugs to relieve acute narcotic withdrawal symptoms
    II.   administer drugs to relieve acute narcotic withdrawal symptoms
    III.   administer drugs to provide narcotic drug-dependent patients with maintenance treatment
    (A) I only   (B) III only   (C) I & II only
    (D) II & III only   (E) I, II, & III

187.   Which of the following is true of DEA Form 222?
    I.   May be used to transfer Schedule II drugs from one pharmacy to another.
    II.   May be used to return Schedule II drugs to the supplier
    III.   It must contain the name and address of the supplier from whom schedule II controlled substances are being ordered.
    (A) I only   (B) III only   (C) I & II only
    (D) II & III only   (E) I, II, & III

188.   Oral orders for Schedule II drugs may be accepted and dispensed by a pharmacist
    I.   in an emergency situation.
    II.   if the physician is more than 100 miles away from the pharmacy.
    III.   if a patient is a regular customer of the pharmacy.
    (A) I only   (B) III only   (C) I & II only
    (D) II & III only   (E) I, II, & III

189.   Schedule II prescriptions
    I.   may only be refilled once
    II.   may be partially filled under certain conditions
    III.   written for a hospice patient may be faxed to a pharmacy
    (A) I only   (B) III only   (C) I & II only
    (D) II & III only   (E) I, II, & III

190. A pharmacist may partially fill a Schedule II prescription
    I.   and the remaining portion of the prescription
         may be filled within 72 hr of the partial fill.
    II. if the pharmacist does not have enough
         medication in stock to completely fill the
         prescription.
    III. if the patient only wants some of the
         medication prescribed.
    (A) I only   (B) III only   (C) I & II only
    (D) II & III only (E) I, II, & III

191. A faxed Schedule II prescription from the prescriber
    to a pharmacy is permitted
    I.   at any time as long as it is followed by a written
         "cover" prescription.
    II. if the patient is a resident of a Long Term Care
         Facility
    III. if the patient is a hospice patient.
    (A) I only   (B) III only   (C) I & II only
    (D) II & III only (E) I, II, & III

192. To be admitted to a comprehensive maintenance
    program, a narcotic-dependent individual must have
    been physiologically dependent on narcotics for at
    least
    (A) 30 days   (B) 90 days   (C) 180 days
    (D) 12 months (E) 18 months

193. Which of the following is/are NOT required to be on
    a prescription for a controlled substance?
    I.   DEA number of the practitioner
    II. The date on which the prescription was signed
    III. The date of birth of the patient
    (A) I only   (B) III only   (C) I & II only
    (D) II & III only (E) I, II, & III

194.   Which of the following is true?
I.   Original schedule III, IV, or V prescriptions may be transferred from one pharmacy to another for the purpose of refill dispensing.
II.   Information from schedule III, IV, or V prescriptions may not be transferred to another pharmacy unless authorized by the prescriber to do so.
III.   Pharmacies electronically sharing a real-time, online database may transfer refills to one another as long as the number of refills transferred does not exceed those authorized by the prescriber or the law.
(A) I only   (B) III only   (C) I & II only
(D) II & III only   (E) I, II, & III

195.   Which of the following drug products must be purchased by pharmacies using DEA Form 222?
I.   Ritalin
II.   MS Contin
III.   Dalgan
(A) I only   (B) III only   (C) I & II only
(D) II & III only   (E) I, II, & III

196.   Which of the following is NOT required on the prescription label when the pharmacist fills a controlled substance prescription?
I.   Date of initial filling
II.   Federal "Caution" warning
III.   Number of dosage units dispensed
(A) I only   (B) III only   (C) I & II only
(D) II & III only   (E) I, II, & III

197. Which of the following is true of Schedule II controlled substances?
    I. They may be dispensed by a community pharmacist only pursuant to a written prescription signed by the practitioner.
    II. They may be administered or dispensed by a physician without a prescription to a patient with chronic pain.
    III. They may be administered by an institutional pharmacist pursuant to an order for immediate administration to the ultimate user.
    (A) I only   (B) III only   (C) I & II only
    (D) II & III only   (E) I, II, & III

198. Which of the following is true of controlled substance inventories?
    I. Inventories for schedule II controlled substances must be kept separately from all other records of the pharmacy.
    II. Controlled substance inventories must be performed annually.
    III. The registrant must keep inventory records for at least 5 years from the date performed.
    (A) I only   (B) III only   (C) I & II only
    (D) II & III only   (E) I, II, & III

199. Short-term narcotic detoxification is defined as treatment that is for a period of less than
    (A) 30 days   (B) 60 days   (C) 90 days
    (D) 180 days   (E) 1 year

200. Which of the following types of products in a hospital pharmacy must be bar-coded?
    I. prescription drugs
    II. biologicals
    III. nonprescription drugs
    (A) I only   (B) III only   (C) I & II only
    (D) II & III only   (E) I, II, & III

201.   The statement "Rx only" does NOT need to appear on the packaging of
(A)   orphan drugs
(B)   controlled substances
(C)   legend drugs
(D)   OTC products
(E)   injectable products

202.   Who is responsible for the retrospective drug utilization reviews established by OBRA 90?
(A)   all dispensing pharmacists
(B)   consultant pharmacists
(C)   each state
(D)   hospital pharmacies
(E)   individual community pharmacies

203.   Which of the following statements is (are) true with respect to the National Drug Code?
I.   NDC must be imprinted on tablets.
II.   NDC must be imprinted on capsules.
III.   All prescription drug products marketed in the US must have NDC's.
(A) I only   (B) III only   (C) I & II only
(D) II & III only   (E) I, II, & III

204.   When a physician faxes a Schedule II prescription to a pharmacy for a LTCF patient
I.   the pharmacist must call the LTCF to verify the identity of the patient.
II.   the physician must first call the pharmacy to advise them that a fax is being issued.
III.   the original written, signed prescription must be presented to the pharmacist for review prior to the actual dispensing of the controlled fax.
(A) I only   (B) III only   (C) I & II only
(D) II & III only   (E) I, II, & III

205. Controlled substance inventories
I.   may be done at any time during the workday.
II.   must be taken at least once each year.
III.   must be made for each registered location.
(A) I only   (B) III only   (C) I & II only
(D) II & III only   (E) I, II, & III

206. A hospital pharmacy director is informed that an employee has been convicted of selling cocaine on the street. Which of the following actions may the director take based upon the Federal Anti-drug Abuse Act of 1988?
I.   warn the employee not to possess or sell illegal drugs in the future
II.   place a letter of reprimand in the employee's personnel file
III.   terminate the employment of the individual
(A) I only   (B) III only   (C) I & II only
(D) II & III only   (E) I, II, & III

207. Narcotic drugs may be dispensed to treat narcotic dependence in which of the following facilities?
I.   Any institutional pharmacy
II.   Any facility with a DEA certified narcotic treatment counselor
III.   FDA and state approved narcotic treatment programs
(A) I only   (B) III only   (C) I & II only
(D) II & III only   (E) I, II, & III

208. Blood and/or urine tests are frequently performed on participants in comprehensive narcotic maintenance treatment programs in order to detect
I.   drug toxicity
II.   hepatotoxicity
III.   continued abuse of drugs
(A) I only   (B) III only   (C) I & II only
(D) II & III only   (E) I, II, & III

209. Which of the following is true?
    I.   Prescribers must keep records of all controlled substances that they dispense directly to the patient.
    II. Prescribers must keep records of all controlled substances administered in the course of narcotic detoxification treatment.
    III. Prescribers must keep records of all controlled substances that they receive as samples
(A) I only   (B) III only   (C) I & II only
(D) II & III only (E) I, II, & III

210. When a patient begins a comprehensive narcotic treatment program, the first day's dose of methadone must generally not exceed
(A) 0.5 mg   (B) 1 mg   (C) 5 mg
(D) 20 mg   (E) 40 mg

211. The use of an FDA approved drug for a use that is not approved for the drug is best described as being:
(A) illegal   (B) off-label   (C) orphan
(D) terminal   (E) unprofessional

212. What acronym is used by the USP to designate sterile products that are prepared in a home infusion pharmacy for delivery to a patient's home residence?
(A) HSD (B) LVP (C) PPI (D) SP (E) TRP

213. Which of the following is/are used in the treatment of narcotic dependence?
    I.   LAAM
    II. methadone
    III. prostigmine
(A) I only   (B) III only   (C) I & II only
(D) II & III only (E) I, II, & III

214. Chloral hydrate is an example of a drug product in controlled substance schedule
(A) I   (B) II   (C) III
(D) IV   (E) V

215. Which of the following products are NOT controlled substances?
I.   Mepergan
II. Melphalan
III. Megestrol acetate
(A) I only   (B) III only   (C) I & II only
(D) II & III only   (E) I, II, & III

216. Prescriptions for which of the following controlled substances may be partially filled upon request of the patient:
I.   Dilaudid
II. Ritalin
III. Empirin w/codeine #4
(A) I only   (B) III only   (C) I & II only
(D) II & III only   (E) I, II, & III

217. Which of the following narcotic-dependent patient groups should NOT generally be given LAAM for their treatment?
I.   Pregnant women
II. Persons under 18 years of age
III. Individuals who are heroin dependent
(A) I only   (B) III only   (C) I & II only
(D) II & III only   (E) I, II, & III

218. Which of the following drug products must be purchased using a DEA Form 222?
I.   Percodan
II. Dilaudid
III. Methadone
(A) I only   (B) III only   (C) I & II only
(D) II & III only   (E) I, II, & III

219. Which of the following drug products are controlled
      substances?
      I.   pemoline (Cylert)
      II   midazolam (Versed)
      III. pimozide (Orap)
      (A) I only   (B) III only   (C) I & II only
      (D) II & III only   (E) I, II, & III

220. Patients treated in an ambulatory care comprehensive
      narcotic treatment program may receive methadone
      doses by which of the following routes?
      I.   oral
      II.   IM
      III. IV
      (A) I only   (B) III only   (C) I & II only
      (D) II & III only   (E) I, II, & III

221. Which of the following drug products must be
      ordered using DEA Form 222?
      I.   Methadone
      II.   Sufentanil
      III. Percocet
      (A) I only   (B) III only   (C) I & II only
      (D) II & III only   (E) I, II, & III

222. Methamphetamine is an example of a drug in controlled
      substance category
      (A) I   (B) II   (C) III
      (D) IV   (E) V

223. The primary objective or charge for individual state
      boards of pharmacy is the
      (A)   protection of individual pharmacists
      (B)   protection of the profession
      (C)   protection of the general public
      (D)   enforcement of federal laws
      (E)   serving as an intermediary between chain,
              independent, and institutional pharmacies

224. HCFA is under the jurisdiction of the
     (A) Attorney General   (B) FDA   (C) HHS
     (D) JCAHO   (E) Dept. of Justice

225. A prescription for methadone is issued for the purpose of managing a patient's narcotic addiction by a physician employed by a narcotic treatment facility. The prescription
     I.   may be filled in most community pharmacies
     II. may be filled only in outpatient institutional pharmacies
     III. may not be filled
     (A) I only   (B) III only   (C) I & II only
     (D) II & III only   (E) I, II, & III

226. Which of the following was the first to require that pharmaceutical manufacturers prove the efficacy of prescription drugs before marketing?
     (A) Durham-Humphrey Amendment (1951)
     (B) F D & C Act of 1938
     (C) Kefauver-Harris Amendment of 1962
     (D) Prescription Drug Marketing Act of 1987
     (E) Pure Food and Drug Act of 1906

227. Which of the following population(s) is(are) covered under the Medicare Modernization Act of 2003?
     I.   Medicare beneficiaries
     II.   Medicaid beneficiaries
     III. Nongovernmental employees.
     (A) I only   (B) III only   (C) I & II only
     (D) II & III only   (E) I, II, & III

228. A drug that is marketed for the treatment of a relatively rare disease is referred to as a(n):
     (A)   me-too drug
     (B)   orphan drug
     (C)   prodrug
     (D)   USAN drug
     (E)   first pass effect drug

229.   The USP/NF is best described as a publication that is published by:
(A)   the HHS
(B)   the FDA
(C)   the Pharmaceutical Manufacturer's Association
(D)   a coalition of US pharmaceutical companies
(E)   an independent organization

230.   A pharmacist dispenses a refill for a prescription that originally was written for Adalat but labels the refill as Procardia. This action may be considered:
(A)   adulteration
(B)   misbranding
(C)   misbranding since the generic name was not included
(D)   proper since the correct drug was dispensed
(E)   negligent only if the prescriber is not informed

231.   Evidence indicates that a marketed drug product may have a new use for another condition. In order to claim this new indication, a drug manufacturer must:
(A)   submit an abbreviated NDA
(B)   submit a supplemental NDA
(C)   submit a NDA
(D)   apply for patent protection
(E)   inform FDA in writing of the revised labeling

232.   A customer had a prescription originally filled on December 1, 2004 and acknowledged receiving the pharmacy's notice of privacy rights under HIPAA. She also receives a refill dispensed on January 2, 2005. What is the earliest date that the pharmacy may discard the patient's acknowledgment?
(A) 12/1/2005   (B) 1/2/2006   (C) 12/1/2010
(D) 1/2/2011   (E) never

233. The advertising to the general public of OTC drugs is basically under the regulatory responsibilities of the:
(A) FDA only   (B) FDA and FTC   (C) FTC only
(D) DEA   (E) HCFA

234. A cosmetic company begins marketing of a facial cream that claims to reverse facial wrinkles. This claim may be legally challenged by the:
(A) FDA only   (B) FDA and FTC   (C) FTC only
(D) DEA   (E) HCFA

235. According to Federal law, a pharmacist must include which of the following on a prescription label?
I.   name of the dispensing pharmacy
II. address of the dispensing pharmacy
III. name of the dispensing pharmacist
(A) I only   (B) III only   (C) I & II only
(D) II & III only   (E) I, II, & III

236. A pharmaceutical company requests the names and addresses of patients who have received a certain antidepressant drug during the past month.
I.   Honoring this request will represent a breach of privacy based upon the Federal Health Insurance Portability and Accountability Act.
II. The request is appropriate if the company only wishes to send the patients information concerning depression.
III. The request may be honored if the company gives the pharmacist an affidavit that a list of the patients' names and addresses will not leave the company.
(A) I only   (B) III only   (C) I & II only
(D) II & III only   (E) I, II, & III

237. Which of the following statements concerning drug recalls is(are) accurate?
I.   They occur only after fatalities have occurred.
II. They can be ordered by the FDA.
III. They are voluntary actions by the pharmaceutical manufacturer
(A) I only   (B) III only   (C) I & II only
(D) II & III only   (E) I, II, & III

238.   Which of the following effervescent products are
        usually exempted from the Poison Prevention Packaging
        Act?
        I.   aspirin
        II.   acetaminophen
        III. potassium chloride
        (A) I only   (B) III only   (C) I & II only
        (D) II & III only   (E) I, II, & III

239.   Federal guidelines indicate that the pharmacist should
        indicate the date on which a prescription refill is dis-
        pensed
        (A)   on the front of the prescription
        (B)   on the back of the prescription
        (C)   on the prescription label
        (D)   in a special refill log book
        (E)   on the counseling sheet given to the patient

240.   Under what circumstance(s) may a pharmacist NOT
        refuse to accept or fill a prescription:
        (A)   The prescription is suspected to be either
               forged or fictitiously written.
        (B)   The patient is known to be HIV positive.
        (C)   The pharmacist believes that he will be
               violating the law by filling the prescription.
        (D)   The drug or drug product is not in stock.
        (E)   The pharmacist believes that the drug product
               may be harmful to the patient.

241.   Which of the following items provided by
        pharmaceutical companies are legal for community
        pharmacies to possess for the dispensing of prescription
        drugs?
        I.   drug samples that are properly labeled
        II.   vouchers intended for filling from the pharmacy's
              stock
        III. starter packs

(A) I only   (B) III only   (C) I & II only
(D) II & III only   (E) I, II, & III

242. Which of the following information must be included in
the bar code of drug products being sold to hospitals?
I. Expiration dates   II. Lot numbers   III. NDC numbers
(A) I only   (B) III only   (C) I & II only
(D) II & III only (E) I, II, & III

243. A physician shares with your pharmacy a topical
moisturizing formula which contains a prescription drug.
Which of the following would be appropriate actions for
your pharmacy to take?
I.   Fill prescriptions written by the physician for 120 g
      of this formula.
II.   Prepare a pound of the formula in anticipation of
      additional prescriptions or refills.
III. Prepare 50 x 120 g of the formula for sale from the
      physician's office.
(A) I only   (B) III only   (C) I & II only
(D) II & III only (E) I, II, & III

244. Which of the following actions is (are) not allowed in a
community pharmacy in respect to prescription drug
samples?
I.   storing
II.   ordering based upon a specific prescriber's request
III. dispensing upon receipt of a prescription
(A) I only   (B) III only   (C) I & II only
(D) II & III only (E) I, II, & III

245. The authority for determining the schedule for a
potentially new controlled substance belongs to the:
(A)   Director of the FDA
(B)   President of the US
(C)   Director of the DEA
(D)   Attorney General of the US
(E)   Director of HHS

246.   Who must be registered with the DEA in order for a
hospitalpharmacy to dispense controlled substances?
I.   the hospital pharmacy
II. the chief pharmacist
III. every pharmacist who dispenses on a regular basis
(A) I only   (B) III only   (C) I & II only
(D) II & III only   (E) I, II, & III

247.   The minimum requirements that a community
pharmacist must follow when filling a controlled
substance prescription written for an outpatient by a
hospital resident is that the
I.   hospital must have a DEA number
II.   resident must have a DEA number
III. drug belongs to either Schedule III or IV
(A) I only   (B) III only   (C) I & II only
(D) II & III only (E) I, II, & III

248.   Based upon federal law, which of the following
schedules of controlled substances may be dispersed
throughout the prescription drug stock of a community
pharmacy?
I.   Schedule II's
II.   Schedule III's
III. Schedule IV and V's
(A) I only   (B) III only   (C) I & II only
(D) II & III only   (E) I, II, & III

249.   When inspecting a chain pharmacy, a DEA inspector
may audit which of the following records?
I.   prescription files
II.   invoices for controlled substances
III. financial records of prescription sales and profits
(A) I only   (B) III only   (C) I & II only
(D) II & III only   (E) I, II, & III

250. Which of the following may a nurse in a doctor's office perform, with the prescriber's permission, with regard to a Schedule III prescription?
   I. write the prescription and sign the prescriber's name
   II. write the prescription except for the drug name, strength, quantity and prescriber's name
   III. write the entire prescription except for signing the prescriber's name
   (A) I only   (B) III only   (C) I & II only
   (D) II & III only   (E) I, II, & III

251. After dispensing prescriptions for several months for a Schedule II analgesic, the pharmacist realizes that the patient with severe pain from bone cancer is addicted to the drug. Which one of the following actions is the most appropriate for the pharmacist?
   (A)   report the situation to the state board of pharmacy
   (B)   report the situation to the state medical board
   (C)   report the situation to the DEA
   (D)   refuse to fill any further prescriptions
   (E)   continue to fill the prescriptions

252. Which one of the following designations for drug products that require a prescription in the United States has replaced the designation "Caution: Federal law prohibits dispensing without a prescription"?
   (A)   "Do not dispense without a prescription."
   (B)   "Do not transfer to a third party."
   (C)   "Federal law prohibits use by anyone other than the original patient."
   (D)   "Rx only"
   (E)   "Legend drug"

253. Which of the following categories of drugs require the above legend?
   I. noncontrolled prescription drugs
   II. Schedule II controlled drugs
   III. Schedule III and IV controlled drugs
   (A) I only   (B) III only   (C) I & II only
   (D) II & III only   (E) I, II, & III

254.   The statement, "Caution: Federal law prohibits the transfer of this drug to any person other than the person for whom it was prescribed" is required on prescription containers for which of the following categories of drugs?
I.   Schedule II
II.   Schedule III
III.   Schedule IV
(A) I only   (B) III only   (C) I & II only
(D) II & III only   (E) I, II, & III

255.   Which of the following are permissible when taking a controlled substance inventory?
I.   assistance of a technician to count tablets
II.   use of a tape recorder
III.   permanent storage of the inventory on a tape recorder
(A) I only   (B) III only   (C) I & II only
(D) II & III only   (E) I, II, & III

256.   Which of the following items must be ordered from a wholesaler on DEA order form 222?
I.   morphine HCl injection 10 mL vials (10 mg/mL)
II.   meperidine HCl tablets 50 mg
III.   diazepam tablets 10 mg
(A) I only   (B) III only   (C) I & II only
(D) II & III only   (E) I, II, & III

257.   The requirement that pharmacists must offer to counsel patients concerning their prescriptions was included in which of the following congressional actions?
(A)   Durham-Humphrey Amendment of 1951
(B)   F,D & C Act of 1938
(C)   Kefauver-Harris Amendment of 1962
(D)   Prescription Drug Marketing Act of 1987
(E)   Omnibus Reconcilation Act of 1990

258. Which of the following actions should a pharmacist take if a patient refuses to be counseled about a new prescription?
    I.   dispense the prescription but inform the prescriber that counseling was refused
    II. refuse to dispense the prescription
    III. dispense the prescription but note in the prescription files that counseling was refused
    (A) I only   (B) III only   (C) I & II only
    (D) II & III only   (E) I, II, & III

259. Which portion of the Federal counseling regulations must be performed by a committee appointed within each individual state?
    I.   retrospective review
    II. prospective review
    III. meta-analysis review
    (A) I only   (B) III only   (C) I & II only
    (D) II & III only   (E) I, II, & III

260. Which of the following is NOT required on the label of unit dose packages prepared in a hospital?
    (A)   name of the drug
    (B)   beyond-use expiration dating
    (C)   manufacturer's expiration date
    (D)   strength of drug
    (E)   control number

261. Which one of the following types of information is useful but not mandatory on the labels of OTC products?
    (A)   name of manufacturer
    (B)   address of manufacturer
    (C)   net contents
    (D)   NDC number
    (E)   adequate directions for use

262. The recent discontinuation of use of
      phenylpropranolamine in OTC products is best described
      as a:
      (A)   Class I recall
      (B)   Class II recall
      (C)   Class III recall
      (D)   mandatory discontinuation
      (E)   voluntary discontinuation

263. Which organization is primarily responsible for
      evaluating the safety and effectiveness of drugs used in
      veterinary practices?
      (A) FDA   (B) FTC   C) SPCA
      (D) humane society   (E) HCFA

264. A pharmacist confides in his hospital's chief pharmacist
      that he has tested positive for HIV. Which of the
      following statements is(are) true?
      I.   The pharmacist may be terminated due to a
            potentially contagious condition
      II.   The pharmacist's access to the preparation of
            parenteral admixtures may be limited.
      III. The pharmacist may be considered disabled under
            the Americans with Disabilities Act.
      (A) I only   (B) III only   (C) I & II only
      (D) II & III only   (E) I, II, & III

265. Which of the following statements on a cranberry extract
      label would be acceptable under DSHEA regulations?
      I.   To reduce E coli counts during a UTI
      II. To reduce the incidence and duration of UTI's
      III. To help maintain a healthy urinary tract in females
      (A) I only   (B) III only   (C) I & II only
      (D) II & III only   (E) I, II, & III

266. Which of the following reference sources depict selected laws and regulations especially for controlled substances?
    (A)   Facts and Comparisons
    (B)   Physician's Desk Reference
    (C)   USP DI Volume I
    (D)   USP DI Volume II
    (E)   USP DI Volume III

267. Which of the following OTC products must be in a tamper-resistant package?
    I.   contact lens solution
    II.   hair shampoo
    III. topical lotion
    (A) I only   (B) III only   (C) I & II only
    (D) II & III only   (E) I, II, & III

268. A prescription is written for Coumadin tablets 5 mg with an indication that substitution is desired. Which of the following manufacturers have suitable products? (see Figure A)
    I.   Bristol Myers Squibb
    II.   Invamed
    III.   Barr
    (A) I only   (B) III only   (C) I & II only
    (D) II & III only   (E) I, II, & III

269. A prescription is written for warfarin tablets 2 mg with an indication that substitution is desired. Which of the following manufacturers have suitable products? (See Figure A)
    I.   Bristol Myers Squibb (BMS)
    II.   Invamed
    III.   Barr
    (A) I only   (B) III only   (C) I & II only
    (D) II & III only   (E) I, II, & III

Figure A

TE Code	RLD	Active Ingredient	Dosage Form; Route	Strength	Proprietary Name	Applicant
AB	No	WARFARIN	Tablet; Oral	1 MG	COUMADIN	BRISTOL MYERS SQUIBB (BMS)
AB	No	WARFARIN	Tablet; Oral	2 MG	COUMADIN	BMS
AB	No	WARFARIN	Tablet; Oral	5 MG	COUMADIN	BMS
AB	Yes	WARFARIN	Tablet; Oral	10 MG	COUMADIN	BMS
AB	No	WARFARIN	Tablet; Oral	2 MG	WARFARIN	BARR
AB	No	WARFARIN	Tablet; Oral	5 MG	WARFARIN	BARR
AB	No	WARFARIN	Tablet; Oral	10 MG	WARFARIN	BARR
AB	No	WARFARIN	Tablet; Oral	2 MG	WARFARIN	INVAMED
AB	No	WARFARIN	Tablet; Oral	5 MG	WARFARIN	INVAMED
AB	No	WARFARIN	Tablet; Oral	10 MG	WARFARIN	INVAMED

270.   In order to be considered bioequivalent with Bristol Myers Squibb's Coumadin tablets, Barr's warfarin sodium tablets must have the same (See Figure A):

I.   color
II.   excipients
III.   drug level

(A) I only   (B) III only   (C) I & II only
(D) II & III only   (E) I, II, & III

271. A prescription calls for Nitro-Dur transdermal patch 0.1 mg/hr. Which of the following transdermal products may be dispensed if substitution is required? (See Figures B & C)
I.   3M's Minitran 0.1 mg/hr.
II.   Mylan's NTG 0.1 mg/hr.
III.   Novartis's NTG 0.1 mg/hr.
(A) I only   (B) III only   (C) I & II only
(D) II & III only   (E) I, II, & III

272. Which of the following companies' 0.2 mg/hr nitroglycerin patches are considered to be interchangeable when substituting? (See Figures B & C)
I.   Hercon Labs
II.   Mylan
III.   Novartis
(A) I only   (B) III only   (C) I & II only
(D) II & III only   (E) I, II, & III

273. A prescription order is written "NTG injection 5 mg/mL". Which of the following statements is(are) true based upon Figure C?
I.   Abbott's product may be used.
II.   Nitroglycerin injection by Novartis may be used.
III.   The AP classification indicates that the products are interchangeable.
(A) I only   (B) III only   (C) I & II only
(D) II & III only   (E) I, II, & III

274. A prescription order is written "NTG transdermal patch 0.4 mg/hr. Do NOT substitute. Which of the following companies' products could the pharmacist dispense?
I.   Novartis
II.   Hercon
III.   Mylan
(A) I only   (B) III only   (C) I & II only
(D) II & III only   (E) I, II, & III

275.   A prescription order is written "Tranderm-Nitro 0.4 mg/hr". Assuming that substitution is NOT permissible, which of the following companies' products could be used? (See Figure C)

    I.   Novartis
    II.   Mylan
    III.   Hercon

    (A) I only   (B) III only   (C) I & II only
    (D) II & III only (E) I, II, & III

276.   A pharmacy carries a complete stock of Nitro-Dur and Minitran patches. In which of the following strengths are these two lines considered bioequivalent? (See Figure B)

    I.   0.2 mg/hr
    II.   0.4 mg/hr
    III.   0.6 mg/hr

    (A) I only   (B) III only   (C) I & II only
    (D) II & III only (E) I, II, & III

277.   Ephedra may no longer be present in which of the following products in a community pharmacy?

    I.   Nonprescription drug products
    II.   Herbal teas
    III.   Dietary supplements

    (A) I only   (B) III only   (C) I & II only
    (D) II & III only (E) I, II, & III

Figure B

TE Code	RLD	Active Ingredient	Dosage Form; Route	Strength	Proprietary Name	Applicant
AB1	Yes	NITROGLYCERIN	Film, Extended Release; Transdermal	0.1 MG/HR	NITRODUR	KEY
AB1	Yes	NITROGLYCERIN		0.2 MG/HR	NITRODUR	KEY
AB1	Yes	NITROGLYCERIN		0.4 MG/HR	NITRODUR	KEY
AB1	Yes	NITROGLYCERIN			NITRODUR	KEY
AB1	Yes	NITROGLYCERIN		0.8 MG/HR	NITRODUR	KEY
AB1	No	NITROGLYCERIN	Film, Extended Release; Transdermall	0.1 MG/HR	MINITRAN	3M
AB1	No	NITROGLYCERIN	Tablet; Oral	0.2 MG/HR	MINITRAN	3M
AB1	No	NITROGLYCERIN	Tablet; Oral	0.4 MG/HR	MINITRAN	3M
AB1	No	NITROGLYCERIN	Tablet; Oral	0.6 MG/HR	MINITRAN	3M

278. Pharmaceutical products employed in which of
the following practice settings must contain bar coding?
 I. Hospitals
 II. Pharmacies
 III. Physician offices
 (A) I only (B) III only (C) I & II only
 (D) II & III only (E) I, II, & III

Figure C

TE Code	RLD	Active Ingredient	Dosage Form; Route	Strength	Proprietary Name	Applicant
AB2	Yes	NITROGLYCERIN	Film, Extended Release; Transdermal	0.1 MG/HR	TRANSDERM-NITRO	NOVARTIS
AB2	Yes	NITROGLYCERIN		0.2 MG/HR	TRANSDERM-NITRO	NOVARTIS
AB2	Yes	NITROGLYCERIN		0.4 MG/HR	TRANSDERM-NITRO	NOVARTIS
AB2	Yes	NITROGLYCERIN		0.6 MG/HR	TRANSDERM-NITRO	NOVARTIS
AB2	No	NITROGLYCERIN		0.2 MG/HR	NITROGLYCERIN	HERCON
AB2	No	NITROGLYCERIN		0.4 MG/HR	NITROGLYCERIN	HERCON
AB2	No	NITROGLYCERIN		0.6 MG/HR	NITROGLYCERIN	HERCON
AB2	No	NITROGLYCERIN		0.1 MG/HR	NITROGLYCERIN	MYLAN
AB2	No	NITROGLYCERIN		0.2 MG/HR	NITROGLYCERIN	MYLAN
AB2	No	NITROGLYCERIN		0.4 MG/HR	NITROGLYCERIN	MYLAN
AB2	No	NITROGLYCERIN		0.6 MG/HR	NITROGLYCERIN	MYLAN
AP	Yes	NITROGLYCERIN	Injectable; Injection	5 MG/mL	NITROGLYCERIN	ABBOTT
AP	Yes	NITROGLYCERIN	Injectable; Injection	5 MG/mL	NITROGLYCERIN	NOVARTIS

279   When conducting a controlled substance inventory, the registrant
  I.   must make an exact count of open containers of Schedule II substances.
  II.   may estimate the count of a Schedule IV substance in an opened container that originally held 500 tablets.
  III. must make an exact count of all controlled substances in sealed, unopened containers.
  (A) I only   (B) III only   (C) I & II only
  (D) II & III only   (E) I, II, & III

280.   According to Federal law, a pharmacist must include which of the following on a prescription label?
  I.   Expiration date from the manufacturer's label
  II.   The name of the manufacturer
  III. A prescription serial number
  (A) I only   (B) III only   (C) I & II only
  (D) II & III only   (E) I, II, & III

281.   The USP/NF classification system used to describe preparation of HSD's (home-use sterile drug products) uses which of the following terminology?
  (A) Category A through E
  (B) Clean rooms 1 through 4
  (C) High volume versus low volume
  (D) Low risk versus high risk
  (E) Sterile versus almost sterile

282.   A DEA form 222a is used
  (A)   to order Schedule II controlled substances
  (B)   to order all controlled substances
  (C)   as a requisition form for Form 222
  (D)   to return unused controlled substances
  (E)   to register a practitioner with DEA

283.   An inspector from the FDA enters your community pharmacy. He/she may issue citations if which of the following are found?
   I.   Drug samples being sold /dispensed pursuant to a prescription
   II.   Recalled prescription drugs among the drug stock
   III.   Samples stored in the drug stock
   (A) I only   (B) III only   (C) I & II only
   (D) II & III only   (E) I, II, & III

284.   Which of the following actions is (are) permissible under the FDA rules for prescription compounding by pharmacies?
   I.   Advertising to dermatologists that the pharmacy can compound topical antifungal ointments
   II.   Sending brochures to nurse practitioners that the pharmacy compounds topical lotions for psoriasis
   III.   Informing an allergist that the pharmacy can economically compound 50 mg diphenhydramine capsules
   (A) I only   (B) III only   (C) I & II only
   (D) II & III only   (E) I, II, & III

285.   In which of the following situations are child-resistant closures NOT required?
   I.   When a community pharmacist dispenses fewer than 10 tablets of a drug product
   II.   When a hospital pharmacy is filling a prescription for an outpatient
   III.   When a hospital pharmacy fills a prescription for an inpatient
   (A) I only   (B) III only   (C) I & II only
   (D) II & III only   (E) I, II, & III

286. The organization responsible for the accreditation of
many health institutions such as hospitals is the:
(A) APhA   (B) ASHP   (C) HHS
(D) FTC   (E) JCAHO

287. A pharmacy providing services under the Medicare
Modernization Act of 2003, that uses the program's
discount cards, may establish a formulary limiting the
drugs to which of the following?
(A)   the top 200 frequently dispensed drugs
(B)   only drugs available generically
(C)   only brand-name drugs
(D)   100 brand-name drugs plus their equivalent
        generic products
(E)   at least one drug from each of 208 therapeutic
        categories

288. Therapeutic substitution is allowed only if an institution
is:
(A) nonprofit
(B) for profit
(C) licensed to do so
(D) using a formulary system
(E) under the supervision of a PharmD

289. The Consumer Product Safety Commission is
responsible for which one of the following?
(A) Federal Food, Drug and Cosmetic Act
(B) DSHEA
(C) Prescription drug to OTC status
(D) Poison Prevention Packaging Act
(E) Good Manufacturing Practice program

290. For which one of the following drugs must a patient sign
an informed consent before receiving an original
prescription?
(A) isotretinoin   (B) morphine sulfate, sust. release
(C) paroxetine   (D) sumatriptan   (E) vancomycin

291.   Which of the following are Schedule II controlled
        substances?
        I.   morphine
        II.   fentanyl
        III. secobarbital
        (A) I only   (B) III only   (C) I & II only
        (D) II & III only   (E) I, II, & III

292.   How frequently may a patient with a Medicare-endorsed
        discount card change his/her provider?
        (A) every month
        (B) every 6 months
        (C) once a year
        (D) whenever he/she desires
        (E) never

Answers to Sample Questions

1. E	31. E	61. E	91. C
2. C	32. C	62. A	92. B
3. B	33. B	63. A	93. A
4. C	34. D	64. D	94. A
5. C	35. B	65. C	95. A
6. C	36. B	66. B	96. B
7. D	37. A	67. A	97. A
8. B	38. C	68. E	98. D
9. A	39. B	69. E	99. A
10. E	40. E	70. B	100. A
11. C	41. D	71. C	101. C
12. D	42. B	72. D	102. E
13. C	43. C	73. C	103. B
14. C	44. C	74. D	104. B
15. E	45. C	75. B	105. D
16. A	46. A	76. E	106. B
17. C	47. C	77. B	107. C
18. E	48. B	78. B	108. D
19. A	49. D	79. A	109. A
20. B	50. D	80. B	110. C
21. E	51. E	81. D	111. A
22. C	52. C	82. E	112. B
23. C	53. D	83. C	113. D
24. A	54. C	84. D	114. C
25. C	55. C	85. B	115. A
26. A	56. C	86. B	116. C
27. B	57. B	87. E	117. C
28. B	58. D	88. E	118. D
29. D	59. C	89. D	119. B
30. C	60. C	90. D	120. C

121. B	151. D	181. A	211. B
122. C	152. D	182. C	212. A
123. A	153. A	183. B	213. C
124. C	154. E	184. E	214. D
125. C	155. B	185. E	215. D
126. C	156. B	186. C	216. B
127. E	157. B	187. E	217. C
128. D	158. C	188. A	218. E
129. A	159. E	189. D	219. C
130. C	160. C	190. C	220. A
131. C	161. A	191. D	221. E
132. A	162. B	192. D	222. B
133. C	163. C	193. B	223. C
134. A	164. A	194. B	224. C
135. A	165. C	195. C	225. B
136. C	166. B	196. B	226. C
137. A	167. D	197. E	227. A
138. B	168. A	198. A	228. B
139. C	169. C	199. A	229. E
140. E	170. A	200. E	230. B
141. A	171. B	201. D	231. B
142. A	172. A	202. C	232. C
143. A	173. E	203. B	233. C
144. C	174. E	204. B	234. B
145. C	175. D	205. B	235. C
146. E	176. C	206. E	236. A
147. D	177. C	207. B	237. B
148. D	178. D	208. B	238. E
149. A	179. D	209. C	239. B
150. A	180. C	210. E	240. B

241. D	254. E	267. A	280. B
242. B	255. C	268. D	281. D
243. C	256. C	269. E	282. C
244. E	257. E	270. B	283. E
245. D	258. B	271. A	284. C
246. A	259. A	272. E	285. B
247. A	260. C	273. E	286. E
248. E	261. D	274. E	287. E
249. C	262. E	275. A	288. D
250. B	263. A	276. E	289. D
251. E	264. B	277. B	290. A
252. D	265. B	278. A	291. E
253. E	266. E	279. E.	292. C

Section N

U.S. Boards of Pharmacy

Alabama State Board of Pharmacy
Jerry Moore, Exec. Dir.
1 Perimeter Park South
Suite 425 S
Birmingham, AL 35243
205/967-0130
www.albop.com

Alaska Board of Pharmacy
Sher Zinn
Licensing Examiner
PO Box 110806
Juneau, AK 99811-0806
907/465-2589
www.dced.state.ak.us/occ/ppha.htm

Arizona State Board of Pharmacy
Harlan Wand
Executive Director
4425 W. Olive Avenue, Suite 140
Glendale, AZ 85302
623/463-2727
www.pharmacy.state.az.us

Arkansas State Board of Pharmacy
Charles S. Campbell
Executive Director
101 E. Capitol, Suite 218,
Little Rock, AR 72201
501/682-0190
www.state.ar.us/asbp

California State Board of Pharmacy
Patricia F. Harris, Executive Officer
400 R Street, Suite 4070
Sacramento, CA 95814
916/445-5014
www.pharmacy.ca.gov

Colorado State Board of Pharmacy
Susan L. Warren
Program Director
1560 Broadway, Suite 1350
Denver, CO 80202-5143
303/894-7800
www.dora.state.co.us/pharmacy

Connecticut Commission of Pharmacy
Michelle Sylvestre, Board Administrator
State Office Building, 165 Capitol Avenue, Room 147
Hartford, CT 06106
860/713-6070
www.ctdrugcontrol.com/rxcommision.htm

Delaware State Board of Pharmacy
David W. Dryden
Executive Secretary
P.O. Box 637
Dover, DE 19903
302/744-4547
www.professionallicensing.state.de.us

District of Columbia Board of Pharmacy
Bonnie Rampersaud,
Executive Director
825 N. Capitol St, N.E., 2nd Floor
Washington, DC 20002
202/442-4767

Florida Board of Pharmacy
Danna Droz
Executive Director
4052 Bald Cypress Way, Bin #CO4
Tallahassee, FL 32399-3254
850/250-4292
www.doh.state.fl.us/mqa

Georgia State Board of Pharmacy
Sylvia L. Bond, Executive Director
237 Coliseum Drive
Macon, GA 31217-3858
478/207-1640
www.sos.state.ga.us/plb/pharmacy

Guam Board of Examiners for Pharmacy
Teresita Villagomez, Acting Administrator
P.O. Box 2816
Hagatna, GU 96932
671/735-7406

Hawaii State Board of Pharmacy
Lee Ann Teshima, Executive Officer
P.O. Box 3469
Honolulu, HI 96801
808/586-2694
www.state.hi.us/dcca/pvl/

Idaho Board of Pharmacy
Richard Markuson, Executive Director
3380 American Terr, Suite 320
Boise, ID 83706
208/334-2356
www.accessidaho.org/bop/

Illinois State Board of Pharmacy
Alicia Purchase, Pharmacy Coordinator
320 W. Washington Street, 3rd Fl.
Springfield, IL 62786
217/782-8556
www.dpr.state.il.us/

Indiana Board of Pharmacy
Joshua Bolin, Director
402 W. Washington Street, Room W066
Indianapolis, IN 46204-2739
317/234-2067
www.in.gov/hpb/boards/isbp/

Iowa Board of Pharmacy Examiners
Lloyd K. Jessen
Executive Secretary/Director
400 SW Eighth St, Suite E
Des Moines, IA 50309-4688
515/281-5944
www.state.ia.us/ibpe

Kansas State Board of Pharmacy
Debra Billingsley, Executive Secretary/Director
Landon State Office Building
900 Jackson, Room 560
Topeka, KS 66612-1231
785/296-4056
www.accesskansas.org/pharmacy

Kentucky Board of Pharmacy
Jeffrey Osman, Acting Executive Director
23 Millcreek Park
Frankfort, KY 40601-9230
502/573-1580
 www.state.ky.us/boards/pharmacy/

Louisiana Board of Pharmacy
Malcolm J. Broussard
Executive Director
5615 Corporate Blvd., Suite 8E,
Baton Rouge, LA 70808-2537
225/925-6496
www.labp.com

Maine Board of Pharmacy
Geraldine Betts
Board Administrator
35 State House Station
Augusta, ME 04333
207/624-8620
www.maineprofessionalreg.org

Maryland Board of Pharmacy
LaVerne George Naesea, Executive Director
4201 Patterson Avenue
Baltimore, MD 21215-2299
410/764-4755
www.dhmh.state.md.us/pharmacyboard/

Massachusetts Board of Registration in Pharmacy
Charles R. Young
Executive Director
239 Causeway Street, Suite 500
Boston, MA 02114
617/727-9953
www.mass.gov/dpl/boards/ph/index.htm

Michigan Board of Pharmacy
Ann Marie Pischea
Licensing Division
611 W. Ottawa, 1st Fl.
P.O. Box 30670
Lansing, MI 48909-8170
517/335-0918
www.cis.state.mi.us

Minnesota Board of Pharmacy
David E. Holmstrom
Executive Director
2829 University Avenue S.E., Suite 530
Minneapolis, MN 55414-3251
612/617-2201
www.phcybrd.state.mn.us

Mississippi State Board of Pharmacy
Leland McDivitt
Executive Director
204 Key Drive, Suite C
Madison, MS 39110
601/605-9556
www.mbp.state.ms.us

Missouri Board of Pharmacy
Kevin E. Kinkade
Executive Director
P.O. Box 625
Jefferson City, MO 65102
573/751-0091
www.pr.mo.gov

Montana Board of Pharmacy
Rebecca Deschamps, RPh, Executive Director
P.O. Box 200513
301 S. Park Ave, 4th Floor
Helena, MT 59620-0513
406/841-2356
www.discoveringmontana.com

Nebraska Board of Examiners in Pharmacy
Becky Wisell, Executive Secretary
P.O. Box 94986
Lincoln, NE 68509
402/471-2115
www.hhs.state.ne.us

Nevada Board of Pharmacy
Keith W. Macdonald
Executive Secretary
555 Double Eagle Court, Suite 1100
Reno, NV 89521
775/850-1440
www.state.nv.us/pharmacy/

New Hampshire Board of Pharmacy
Paul G. Boisseau
Executive Secretary
57 Regional Drive, Concord, NH 03301-8518
603/271-2350
www.state.nh.us/pharmacy/

New Jersey State Board of Pharmacy
Joanne Boyer
Executive Director
124 Halsey Street
Newark, NJ 07102
973/504-6450
www.state.nj.us/lps/ca/brief/pharm.htm

New Mexico Board of Pharmacy
Jerry Montoya, Chief Inspector/Director
5200 Oakland NE, Suite A
Albuquerque, NM 87113
505/222-9830
www.state.nm.us/pharmacy

New York Board of Pharmacy
Lawrence Mokhiber, Exec. Secy.
89 Washington Avenue, 2nd Floor West
Albany, NY 12234-1000
518/474-3817 ext. 130
www.op.nysed.gov/pharm.htm

North Carolina Board of Pharmacy
David R. Work
Executive Director
P.O. Box 4560
Chapel Hill, NC 27515-4560
919/942-4454
www.ncbop.org

North Dakota State Board of Pharmacy
Howard C. Anderson, Jr.
Executive Director
P.O. Box 1354
Bismarck, ND 58502-1354
701/328-9535
www.nodakpharmacy.com

Ohio State Board of Pharmacy
William T. Winsley
Executive Director
77 S. High Street, Room 1702
Columbus, OH 43215-6126
614/466-4143
www.pharmacy.ohio.gov

Oklahoma State Board of Pharmacy
Bryan H. Potter
Executive Director
4545 Lincoln Blvd., Suite 112
Oklahoma City, OK 73105-3488
405/521-3815
www.pharmacy.state.ok.us

Oregon State Board of Pharmacy
Gary A. Schnabel, Executive Director
800 N.E. Oregon Street - #9
State Office Bldg., Room 425
Portland, OR 97232
503/731-4032
www.pharmacy.state.or.us

Pennsylvania State Board of Pharmacy
Melanie Zimmerman, Executive Secretary
124 Pine Street
P.O. Box 2649
Harrisburg, PA 17105-2649
717/783-7156
www.dos.state.pa.us/bpoa/phabd/mainpage.htm

Puerto Rico Board of Pharmacy
Magda Bouet Graña
Executive Director
Call Box 10200
Santruce, PR 00908
787/725-8161

Rhode Island Board of Pharmacy
Catherine A. Cordy
Chief of the Board
3 Capitol Hill, Room 205
Providence, RI 02908
401/222-2837
www.health.state.ri.us/hsr/pharmacy.htm

South Carolina Board of Pharmacy
LeeAnn Bundrick
Administrator
110 Centerview Drive, Suite 306
Columbia, SC 29211-1927
803/896-4700
www.llr.state.sc.us/pol/pharmacy

South Dakota State Board of Pharmacy
Dennis M. Jones
Executive Secretary
4305 S. Louise Ave., Suite 104
Sioux Falls, SD 57106
605/362-2737
www.state.sd.us/doh/pharmacy

Tennessee Board of Pharmacy
Kendall M. Lynch, Director
Davy Crockett Tower, Second Floor
500 James Robertson Parkway
Nashville, TN 37243
615/741-2718
www.state.tn.us/commerce/boards/pharmacy

Texas State Board of Pharmacy
Gay Dodson, Executive Director
333 Guadalupe, Tower 3
Suite 600, Box 21
Austin, TX 78701-3942
512/305-8000
www.tsbp.state.tx.us

Utah Board of Pharmacy
Diana L. Baker, Bureau Director
160 E. 300 South, P.O. Box 146741
Salt Lake City, UT 84114-6741
801/530-6719
www.dopl.utah.gov/

Vermont Board of Pharmacy
Peggy Atkins, Board Administrator
26 Terrace Street, Drawer 09
Montpelier, VT 05609-1106
802/828-2875
www.vtprofessionals.org/opr1/pharmacists/

Virginia Board of Pharmacy
Elizabeth Scott Russell
Executive Director
6606 W. Broad Street, 5th Floor
Richmond, VA 23230-1712
804/662-9911
www.dhp.state.va.us/pharmacy/default.htm

Virgin Islands Board of Pharmacy
Lydia T. Scott, Executive Assistant
Roy L. Schneider Hospital, 48 Sugar Estate,
St. Thomas, VI 00802
340/774-0117

Washington State Board of Pharmacy
Steven M. Saxe, Executive Director
P.O. Box 47863
Olympia, WA 98504-7863
360/236-4825
www.doh.wa.gov

West Virginia Board of Pharmacy
William T. Douglass, Jr., Executive Director
232 Capitol Street
Charleston, WV 25301
304/558-0558
www.wvbop.com/

Wisconsin Pharmacy Examining Board
Tom Ryan, Bureau Director
1400 E. Washington, P.O. Box 8935
Madison, WI 53708
608/266-2811
http://drl.wi.gov/prof/phar/def.htm

Wyoming State Board of Pharmacy
James T. Carder
Executive Director
632 S. David Street
Casper, WY 82601
307/234-0294
http://pharmacyboard.state.wy.us/

Index

D

T

U

V

W

X

NOTE PAGE

NOTE PAGE

NOTE PAGE

NOTE PAGE

NOTE PAGE

NOTE PAGE

NOTE PAGE

NOTE PAGE

NOTE PAGE

NOTE PAGE

NOTE PAGE

NOTE PAGE

NOTE PAGE

NOTE PAGE